A Breath of Hope: Early Detection of Lung Disease

Kry

Table of Contents

1. Introduction

The following book is divided into five chapters: Chapter 1 provides background into obstructive lung disease, the implications of undiagnosed lung disease, a rationale for a case-finding tool, and the study objectives. Chapter 2 presents the study methodology for the derivation of the questionnaire. Chapter 3 presents the results of the model, including prospective external validation and prospective reliability assessment. Chapter 4 summarizes the findings, strengths, limitations, and future directions. Chapter 5 presents the conclusions of the book.

1.1   Background

In 2017, the Global Lancet reported 545 million people were living with a chronic respiratory disease.[1] The prevalence of chronic respiratory diseases have increased by almost 40% in the last 30 years and, to date, they are the third leading cause of death in the world.[1] Of the chronic respiratory disease cases worldwide, chronic obstructive pulmonary disease (COPD) and asthma are the most common.[1,2] The Global Health Epidemiology Reference Group estimate the current prevalence of COPD as approximately 12% for persons over 30 years of age.[3] Based on a 2002-2003 World Health Survey report, the prevalence of asthma is approximately 4.5% for young adults between the ages of 18 and 45 years.[1,4]

COPD and asthma are both obstructive lung diseases (OLD), referring to disorders hallmarked by airflow limitation.[5] According to the Global Initiative for Asthma (GINA), asthma is a heterogeneous disease and defined as a chronic inflammation of the airways.[6] Based on the Global Initiative for Chronic Obstructive Lung Disease (GOLD), COPD is defined as a "common, preventable, treatable disease… characterized by persistent respiratory symptoms and airflow limitation that is due to airway and/or alveolar abnormalities…caused by exposure to noxious particles or gases."[7] Both disorders have distinct clinical presentations and natural disease progression.[8] However, as reported by GOLD and GINA, both disorders can overlap in clinical characteristics and symptoms.[6,7,9] In most cases, asthma presents during childhood; however, its onset can occur at any age, and is reversible spontaneously or following treatment.[6]

Although the natural history of disease progression for asthma is variable and difficult to predict for each individual, severe disease progression is relatively rare among all age groups. In comparison, COPD tends to appear during middle age, progressively worsens with advancing age, and is only partially reversible.[10]

1.2   Etiology
1.2.1   Chronic Obstructive Pulmonary Disease

Tobacco smoke is the most significant etiological factor for COPD: the adverse effects of lung decline from smoking have been well-documented along with the increased likelihood of disease-onset compared to non-smokers.[11–14] Approximately 90% of chronic lung diseases cases are cigarette smokers, and smokers experience more lung abnormalities and higher mortality rates compared to non-smokers.[15] However, the effects of smoking cessation are still advantageous even for long-term smokers.[16,17] Research in patients with early COPD has demonstrated that cigarette smoking is inversely associated with rapid decline in lung function, measured by forced expiratory volume in the first second (FEV_1).[11,18] Reduced FEV_1 is associated with increased risk of developing chronic lung disease and other diseases, including stroke and lung cancer.[19] Given that the FEV_1 is a biomarker for premature morbidity and mortality, smoking cessation is regarded as a highly effective method to preserve lung function and slow disease progression. A prospective 8-year study by Fletcher and Peto found the rate of FEV_1 decline can revert to normal after quitting smoking.[11] The 1994 Lung Health Study was another study assessing the effects of smoking status on rate of decline in lung function (measured by the rate of decline in FEV_1).[16] Compared to sustained quitters and intermediate quitters, continuous smokers experienced a faster rate of decline in lung function over a 10-year period and they experienced a higher rate of self-reported lower respiratory illnesses. Overall, quitting smoking reduced the rate of respiratory illnesses and, in turn, reduced additional loss of lung function.

The adverse effects of smoking exposure are not solely limited to cigarettes. For instance, long-term exposures to indoor air pollution (e.g., biomass fuels) and outdoor air pollution (e.g., traffic-related) are associated with increased risk.[20,21] Maternal smoking and second-hand smoking are other risk factors for developing chronic respiratory symptoms.[22]

Despite the strength of evidence against tobacco smoke, not all smokers will develop COPD.[14,23] Given the variability of disease-onset among smokers, other factors, including a genetic predisposition, being male, childhood respiratory-tract infections, and occupational exposures can influence risk.[24-27]

1.2.2   Asthma

The underlying pathophysiology of disease-onset for asthma remains unclear, but research has associated complex gene-environmental interactions occurring in early life and in utero as risks for development of asthma. Hereditary factors, prenatal factors (e.g., premature birth, caesarian delivery, diet, maternal smoking) and environmental factors (e.g., allergens, microbes, antibiotics, outdoor air pollution) are the most robust risk predictors.[28-35] Prenatal maternal smoking and passive exposure have shown consistent associations to adverse wheezing symptoms and physician-diagnosed asthma.[28-30] Findings from a systematic review and meta-analysis, reviewing 79 prospective studies, found an 85% increased odds of incident asthma in children exposed to prenatal maternal smoking.[29] Exposure to certain environmental factors, including dust mites, cockroach allergens, and pollen have been associated with increased asthma.[36-38] However, the relationship between animal exposure and risk have varied. Among two prospective cohorts and a case-control study, a greater risk from exposure to dogs, farm animals, and cats was shown[39-41] while two retrospective birth cohorts and a case-control study found a reduced risk, or rather a protective effect, from dogs and farm animals.[42-45] Moreover, children exposed to wheezing-induced viral respiratory infections, such as rhinoviruses, respiratory syncytial viruses, during early life are predisposed to a higher risk later in life.[46,47] A prospective, six-year study following 289 newborns found infants diagnosed with rhinovirus-induced wheezing in the first three years of life had a 10-fold increased risk of developing asthma at age six[46] For adult-onset asthma, the pathogenesis and the risk factors are less known compared to childhood-onset.[48,49] Adult-onset asthma is reported to have a poorer prognosis than childhood-onset, and is associated with a rapid lung decline and more severe symptoms.[49,50]

Current research suggests severe childhood asthma, obesity, and occupational exposures (e.g., organic solvents, animal-derived chemicals) can influence the development or remission of asthma during adulthood.[51]

1.3 Epidemiology and Cost of Obstructive Lung Disease

Based on the latest Canadian Chronic Disease Surveillance System report, the age-standardized prevalence of physician-diagnosed COPD for persons over 35 years of age was 9.4% in 2012. According to Statistics Canada, the prevalence of physician-diagnosed asthma was 8.1% for persons over 12 years of age in 2014.[52,53] Chronic respiratory diseases account for 4.7% of the global disability-adjusted life years, with COPD accounting for 2.6% and asthma accounting for 1% of the total.[54,55] These estimates illustrate the non-fatal (e.g., morbidity) and fatal burden of asthma and COPD, as disability-adjusted life years represent the number of 'healthy' life years lost from premature death or disability.[54] Global estimates indicate COPD is responsible for more than a million deaths per year with a projection of five million deaths per year by 2060.[7]

The economic burden of these two disorders varies between countries, however the trend of increasing costs remains consistent.[56,57] In the United States, the combined indirect and direct costs of chronic respiratory diseases, in 2016, were $170 billion and more than $9 billion in Canada in 2010.[58–60] Across the globe, and in North America, indirect and direct costs are related to emergency admissions, hospital stays, prescription medications, early retirement, and absenteeism from work.[57] Chapman et al. conducted a 2003 national survey study to determine the costs incurred from COPD in Canada.[61] The total (indirect and direct) annual costs was $3,196 per patient (direct costs were $1,998 per patient and indirect costs were $1,198 per patient). Most indirect costs were attributed to lost days from work while direct costs were primarily from unscheduled visits, such as emergency admissions and inpatient stays.[61] In a 10-year retrospective Canadian matched cohort study by Tavakoli et al. for persons aged 5 to 55 years with asthma, the total annual direct cost was $2,217 per patient with the majority of costs related to medications.[62] Compared to a matched healthy control, a person with physician-diagnosed asthma spent $1,028 more, on average, in costs related to medications, hospitalizations, and outpatient visits.[62]

1.4 Gold Standard for Clinical Diagnosis

Both the GOLD and GINA recommend spirometry as the standard test for a clinical diagnosis of asthma or COPD.[6,7] Spirometry uses the forced vital capacity (FVC) maneuver, a simple and common procedure where a person quickly and forcefully exhales all the air from their lungs after maximum inhalation.[5] The FVC measures the volume exhaled after the maneuver, and alongside the FVC is the FEV_1 (volume of air expelled in the first second of the maneuver) and FEV_1/FVC ratio.[5] The FEV_1/FVC ratio is a significant measure to identify a person with obstructive lung disease, and differentiate between restrictive and obstructive patterns.

Based on GOLD guidelines, a clinical diagnosis for COPD is based on a post-bronchodilator FEV_1/FVC of less than 0.70.[7] This ratio, however, has been recommended by GOLD to be evaluated with a reference standard for the same anthropometric characteristics (i.e., sex, age, race, height) to prevent overdiagnosis, particularly in the elderly.[7,63] Given that lung physiology changes with age (e.g., decreased elasticity), specific parameters (i.e., FEV_1) tend to decline which can lead to a false-positive diagnosis.[63–65] Instead of a fixed criterion, a FEV_1/FVC less than the lower limit of normal, defined as the lower 5th percentile (1.65 standard deviations from the mean) of the reference population, has been proposed. Without the evidence from longitudinal findings, however, evidence-based reviews and GOLD suggests neither one criterion is superior to the other for diagnosis.[5,7,63,66] By comparison, a clinical diagnosis of asthma can be based on a positive bronchodilator reversibility test. This test refers to the administration of a bronchodilator (a medication relaxing the smooth muscles of the airways). Following administration, any increase in FEV_1 of more than 12% and 200mL from the baseline FEV_1 is indicative of reversible, expiratory airflow limitation.[6] A post-bronchodilation measure is used to discriminate between reversible (i.e., asthma) and irreversible (i.e., COPD) airflow limitation and to avoid misclassification.[5,67,68] In particular, a post-bronchodilator FEV_1/FVC less than 0.70 would indicate COPD; however, changes in the FEV_1 greater than 12% and 200mL would suggest asthma.

According to the GOLD report, with proper calibration, correct interpretation of readings and reference equations, and adequate patient performance, high quality spirometry readings in any healthcare setting is possible.[7] Adherence to guidelines in the 2005 American Thoracic Society (ATS) and the European Respiratory Society (ERS) Task Force: Standardisation of Lung Function Testing can ensure reproducible and acceptable results.[69]

1.5   Statement of Issue

Undiagnosed asthma and COPD (henceforth referred to collectively as obstructive lung diseases, OLD) remains a prevalent health issue in Canada and in other countries.[7,54,70–75] The current global and Canadian prevalence rates for reported OLD do not reflect the true prevalence of OLD since undiagnosed cases remain missed and uncounted. In a review of four epidemiological surveys from 27 countries, Lamprecht et al. found 81% of the participants, who had met the criteria for spirometry-defined obstructive airflow, had never been diagnosed.[70] Based on a summary of findings, some estimate approximately 70 to 90% of chronic airflow limitation is undiagnosed.[70,76,77]

Undiagnosed OLD remains a complex and multifold issue. The underuse of spirometry in primary care and varying clinical guidelines are two underlying factors.[76–79] Among qualitative-based interviews with physicians and evidence-based reviews, different reasons affect use of spirometry including insufficient staff training, patient discomfort, limited access, time constraints, and personal beliefs.[77,80–83] Even more, equitable access to spirometry is constrained by costs; in Canada, while fee codes may offset the cost of spirometry tests in most provinces, diagnostic fees can vary.[84] On a global scale, assessment of the true prevalence rates of asthma and COPD are hindered by significant gaps in data available from different countries.[7] A review by Ho et al. reported proper spirometry calibration, performance quality, post-bronchodilator use, interpretation of spirometry readings, and accessibility remain a significant challenge for developing countries.[75] Population-based physician cohort studies in sub-Saharan Africa have reported insufficient access and provision of spirometry equipment in private and public hospitals, primary care clinics, and pharmacies.[85,86]

Personal perception of symptoms, existing comorbidities, age, gender, and quality of life can contribute to under-diagnosis. Previous studies have found a diagnosis of COPD can be missed by existing comorbidities,[75] COPD can be overlooked in younger persons (under 50 years of age),[70] and women are more likely than men to be underdiagnosed in primary care.[87,88] For undiagnosed asthma in older persons, this may be linked to the misconception that asthma only affects children. Depression, social isolation, and physical inactivity have also been linked to underdiagnosis of asthma.[89] For both disorders, decreased awareness of symptoms and underreporting of symptoms during primary care visits are significant factors.[90–92] Respiratory symptoms (e.g., cough, phlegm, shortness of breath) can be mistakenly perceived by patients as a by-product of ageing, level of physical fitness, and cigarette smoking, leading to symptom under-reporting, and hence under-diagnosis of OLD.[93]

1.6   Adverse Impact of Undiagnosed Obstructive Lung Disease

Early diagnosis and management of either disease has the potential to improve health-related quality of life, reduce the progression of lung decline, and reduce hospital admissions.[94,95] Moreover, for cases left untreated, emerging research has shown the association of both diseases with increased mortality risk,[77] higher economic and social costs,[96–98] and impaired quality of life and health status.[99–104]

A cross-sectional study in the United States using the National and Nutritional Examination Surveys (NHANES) found participants with undiagnosed OLD had a higher risk of all-cause mortality in comparison to participants without OLD. However, diagnosed cases of OLD still had a higher risk of all-cause mortality overall.[77] In the Canadian Cohort Obstructive Lung Disease (CanCOLD) study, participants with undiagnosed COPD were found to have similar rates of health services usage (i.e., unscheduled doctor visits, emergency department visits, hospitalizations) compared to participants diagnosed with COPD.[105] Similar to the NHANES and CanCOLD findings, Kostikas et al. and Larsson et al. evaluated the differences between a delayed versus early COPD diagnosis.[97,98] Delayed diagnosis was defined as having three or more registered International Classification of Diseases, 10th Revision (ICD-10) indicators in the last five years before a physician-diagnosis. Those with a delayed diagnosis experienced higher rates of hospital admissions, greater use of steroids and antibiotics for respiratory infections, and higher healthcare costs for two years post-diagnosis.

1.7   Overview of Case-finding Instruments for Obstructive Lung Disease

Screening tests are intended to identify undetected conditions or risk markers of disease in asymptomatic individuals in a population. In contrast to traditional screening measures, case-finding involves actively targeting persons at increased risk of disease.[106,107] This distinction is relevant in relation to the 2016 US Preventive Services Task Force (USPSTF) report, in which the USPSTF recommended against the use of spirometry for asymptomatic COPD patients given that there is no adequate evidence to suggest that early detection (prior to symptoms) alters clinical outcomes.[107,108] However, the USPSTF and other organizations (e.g., example, GOLD) state this recommendation is not applicable to those at-risk and present with symptoms. Rather the USPTSTF encourages active case-finding for patients with risk factors, such as cigarette smoking and occupational exposure.[108] One approach of case-finding is to identify those at-risk before signs and symptoms are manifested. Another case-finding strategy adopted in the Undiagnosed COPD and Asthma Population (UCAP) study was to administer two disease-specific screening tools, the Asthma Screening Questionnaire (ASQ) and COPD-Diagnostic Questionnaire (COPD-DQ), to individuals who have symptoms but have not yet been diagnosed with OLD.

1.6.1   Case-finding Instruments for COPD

With the underuse of spirometry in primary care, case-finding strategies are a practical method to identify individuals with airflow obstruction. To date, the UCAP study is the only study to build a case-finding tool for both disorders.

One other study in 2018 by Badnjevic et al. did combine both disorders, but with the objective of determining the accuracy of their Expert Diagnostic System (EDS) to implement in clinical settings.[109] The EDS was two steps. the first step was classification of disease status based on a seven-item symptom questionnaire. If the probability of disease was greater than 50%, the second step was classification of COPD or asthma using a machine learning algorithm, i.e., artificial neural network and fuzzy logic, and inputting spirometry test parameters of the patient. If the EDS classification is not decisive, additional tests are performed until a decision is made. The seven items asked whether the patient is age over 40 years, experiences problems while exercising or doing low-intensity activities, coughs at night or after waking up, has mucus, high-pitched breathing sounds in the morning, high-pitched breathing sounds at night or while working out, or experiences a choking sensation at rest. The authors report the overall result of the EDS using prospective validation in a 2x2 table. The total enrolled in a prospective validation was 1650, of whom 1495 (91%) had OLD. The positive predictive value (PPV) was 99.86%; negative predictive value (NPV) was 74.27%; sensitivity was 98.45%; and specificity was 98.71%. The authors did note the correct classification rate for the seven-item questionnaire was 95.71% for OLD cases; this, however, was validated in a retrospective dataset. While the application has desirable sensitivity and specificity results, the high PPV values reflect the high prevalence (91%) of disease, and the implementation is only feasible in a clinical setting. The most applicable portion of the EDS to a community-setting is the seven-item symptom-based questionnaire, but the specificity, sensitivity, and area under the receiver operating characteristic curve (AUC) are unknown and it has yet to be externally validated.

Table 1 presents a summary of eight instruments used to case-find or to screen participants for COPD. Of the three retrospective studies, two derived their case-finding instrument from the 1988-1994 National Health and Nutritional Examination Survey (NHANES) cohort.[110,111] The five-item Lung Function Questionnaire (LFQ) derived by Yawn et al. includes questions about age, wheeze, dyspnea, phlegm, and smoking history.[110] The diagnostic criterion for airflow obstruction was based on a pre-bronchodilator FEV_1/FVC of less than 0.70 and a self-reported physician diagnosis. At a score above three, the sensitivity (77.8%) was moderate and the specificity (52.4%) was low. The authors, however, did not report positive predictive value (PPV), negative predictive value (NPV) or 95% confidence intervals. The PPV and NPV are valuable when considering the practical usefulness of screening tools in practice. These metrics determine whether persons testing positive or negative do, in fact, have the disease or not. For studies without published PPV or NPV values, the likelihood ratios (LR) were calculated using the specificity and sensitivity data. Similar to the PPV and NPV, LR are diagnostic measures used to express the change in the odds of disease. Positive likelihood ratio can be understood as the increase in odds of disease when a test is positive, and vice-versa for the negative likelihood ratio.

In comparison to other case-finding studies, the sample size (n=387) used to derive the questions was smaller, and the study is limited by potential misclassification of the sample outcome, i.e., based on a self-reported diagnosis. The "Could It Be COPD?" instrument derived by Calverley et al. includes age, phlegm, cough, breathlessness, and smoking history.[111] The sensitivity reported was 80.8% and the specificity was 62.8%. Despite using the NHANES sample, the authors' sample was limited to the dominant American ethnic groups (African Americans, Caucasians, and Mexican-Americans), potentially limiting the generalizability. In addition, no external validation has been conducted on the questionnaire. For both retrospective studies, the diagnostic criterion was based on a pre-bronchodilator FEV_1/FVC. Given pre-bronchodilator spirometry has been shown to lead to overdiagnosis or misdiagnosis of cases, most studies recommend post-bronchodilator spirometry to rule out the possibility of reversible airflow limitation.[67,68]

The TargetCOPD instrument of Haroon et al. was developed from their 2014 retrospective clinical trial study data.[112] The TargetCOPD was a five-item tool consisting of age, smoking status, dyspnea, use of prescription antibiotics, and prescription of salbutamol. The objective was to implement a risk scoring model in primary care offices using electronic health records data. At a cut-point of 7.5, sensitivity and sensitivity were approximately 69% each, with a low PPV of 14.4% and high NPV of 96.6%. External validation of the TargetCOPD, however, has yet to be conducted to assess its generalizability to other populations.

The remaining five studies were prospective cohort and case-control studies.[113–117] Each had used a diagnostic criterion of a post-bronchodilator FEV_1/FVC below the lower limit of normal or below 0.70. The COPD Diagnostic Questionnaire (COPD-DQ) developed by Price et al. was an eight-item tool including age, body mass index, presence of phlegm in the morning, phlegm during a cold, wheeze, weather-dependent cough, allergies, and pack-years of smoking. The authors intended for the COPD-DQ to be used mainly in a high-risk population, i.e. cigarette smokers, thus participants were recruited if they were current or past smokers with no prior diagnosis of airflow obstruction. Overall, sensitivity and specificity at the lower cut-off showed moderate specificity and low sensitivity. However, external validation of the COPD-DQ has shown poor discrimination between those with and without airflow obstruction.[118,119] In one external study conducted on current and former smokers, the specificity was 54% and 24% for cut-offs 19.5 and 16.5, respectively, and the sensitivity was 66% and 89% for the same respective cut-offs.[118]

The COPD-Population Screener developed by Martinez et al. was a five-item tool which included age, sputum, functional limitations, dyspnea, and smoking history. Despite the moderate sensitivity and specificity results, the study population was not reflective of a general screening population. Some limitations of the study were that participants with a previously self-reported or confirmed physician diagnosis were not excluded, and more than 50% of the spirometry test performed did not adhere to the appropriate ATS/ERS reproducibility or acceptability standards. The overall predictive value was high, but participant recruitment was primarily from pulmonary specialist clinics. Similar to the COPD-DQ, the PUMA study and COPD-Population Screener recruited their participants from primary care settings and pulmonary specialist centres.[115,116] Given the disease prevalence is higher when recruiting from clinics, and given the PPV and NPV are dependent on the prevalence, the findings need to be interpreted within this context. As reported among the authors' limitations, external validation in the general population is required to determine the optimal risk-cut off as these study results have not been examined in different settings, i.e., evaluating the instrument in a different country or in a community setting versus hospital setting.

The CAPTURE study by Martinez et al. derived a five-item questionnaire covering exposure to air pollutants, dust, smoke, and second-hand smoke, tiredness, changes in breathing based on the season, breathlessness, and days of work missed from a cold, bronchitis, or pneumonia.[113] The authors reported high sensitivity and low specificity. However, the sample size (n=346) used to derive the questionnaire was small, and the authors did not report PPV or NPV values. Lastly, the COPD Scale developed by Franco-Marina et al. was a two-item questionnaire, consisting of age and smoking status.[114] The sensitivity was 82% but the specificity was low (47%) with no

PPV or NPV values reported. Smoking and age are the most significant predictors for COPD, but they are also significant predictors for other diseases, such as coronary heart disease. A screening questionnaire with only two predictors and without questions related to symptoms or occupational exposures is likely to capture a large number of people who do not actually have COPD.

The available case-finding instruments are encumbered by several methodological limitations, including the data source as self-reported cases were included, small derivation cohorts, limited accuracy in identifying obstructive airflow, and lack of external validation.

Author, Year	Case-finding Questionnaire	Design	Location	Predictors	Risk cut-off	Sensitivity (%)	Specificity (%)	PPV (%)	NPV (%)	AUC	Limitations
Yawn et al.,[110] 2010	LFQ	Retrospective	USA	Age; smoked for >20 years; phlegm; wheeze; breathlessness	≥ 3	77.8	52.4	1.63*	0.424*	0.65	• Based on pre-bronchodilator spirometry • Small sample size (n=387)
Calverley et al.,[111] 2005	Could It Be COPD?	Retrospective	USA	Age ≥ 40; smoking status and pack-years of cigarette smoking; cough; phlegm; breathlessness	3 & ≥ 35 years old	80.8	62.8	32.7	93.6	--	• No validation performed • Based on pre-bronchodilator spirometry
Haroon et al.,[112] 2017	TargetCOPD	Retrospective	Europe	Age; smoking status; dyspnea; salbutamol; antibiotics	≥ 7.5	68.8	68.8	14.4	96.6	0.74	• Recruitment from primary care • Use of electronic health records data
Price et al.,[117] 2006	COPD-DQ	Prospective	Europe, USA	Age; BMI; smoking; weather-dependent cough; wheeze; phlegm; history of allergies	16.5 19.5	58.4 80.4	77.0 57.5	37.0 30.3	89.0 92.7	0.82	• Recruitment from primary care • Poor external validation; unable to discriminate in a high-risk population
Martinez et al.,[116] 2008	COPD-PS	Prospective	USA	Age; smoking; shortness of breath; phlegm; limitation of activities	≥ 5	84.4	60.7	56.8	86.4	0.81	• Participants recruited from pulmonary specialist centres

Study	Test	Design	Country	Predictors	Cut-off						Limitations
											• Included participants with previously diagnosed airflow obstruction
Varela et al.,[115] 2016	PUMA Study	Prospective	Latin America	Age; sex; smoking; dyspnea; phlegm; cough; previous spirometry	≥5	76.3	69.3	38.5	92.1	0.76	• No validation performed • Participants recruited from primary care clinics
Martinez et al.,[113] 2017	CAPTURE Study	Prospective	USA	Exposure to air pollutants, smoke, second-hand smoke, dust; easily tired; breathing during different seasons; limitation of activities; days of work, school, or activities missed	≥2	95.7	44.4	1.72*	0.097*	0.795	• Small sample size (n=346) • No explicit predictor for cigarette smoking status or age
Franco-Marina et al.,[114] 2014	COPD Scale	Prospective	Mexico	Age; pack-years of cigarette smoking	≥10	82.0	47.0	1.55*	0.383*	0.64	• Screening process with only two predictors • Small sample size (n=542)

LFQ=Lung Function Questionnaire; COPD-DQ=COPD Diagnostic Questionnaire; COPD-PS=COPD Population Screener; PUMA=Prevalence Study and Regular Practice, Diagnosis and Treatment, Among General Practitioners in Populations at Risk of COPD in Latin America; CAPTURE=COPD Assessment in Primary Care to Identify Undiagnosed Respiratory Disease and Exacerbation Risk
*Positive and negative likelihood ratios (LR) calculated based on available study data.

1.6.2   Case-finding Instruments for Asthma

Although a substantial number of case-finding studies have been developed for COPD in the past decade, the case-finding literature for asthma is sparse. Most of the case-finding studies done to date to detect undiagnosed asthma have been conducted in children and adolescents.[120–124] Given that case-finding tools derived from younger populations have not yet been validated in adults, and given the different clinical presentations of adults and children, these tools cannot be assumed to be valid for adults.[125]

Shin et al. developed the Asthma Screening Questionnaire (ASQ) as a clinical tool for diagnosing asthma in 2010.[126] The ASQ is a diagnostic instrument developed for individuals over 18 years of age. The objective of the case-control study was to determine the diagnostic accuracy of the ASQ in distinguishing between asthmatics and non-asthmatics. A total of six questions were derived from commonly asked questions during clinical appointments and recommendations from the National Asthma Education and Prevention Program and the Global Initiative for Asthma. The instrument was administered to 50 participants. The authors found the optimal cut-off as 4 where the sensitivity was 96% and the specificity was 100% along with a PPV of 100% and a 96% NPV. Despite the reported high sensitivity and specificity for the ASQ, the small derivation sample size of 50 participants and the absence of internal and external validation limits its generalizability.

In 2010, Deng et al. developed a model to predict the risk of asthma in adults with the objective of reducing the need for methacholine challenge tests in clinical or epidemiological studies.[127] The authors derived the six-item questionnaire using the 2003-04 Shanghai Women's Asthma and Allergy Study cohort who had completed the International Study of Asthma and Allergies in Childhood (ISAAC) survey. The six items included age, family history of allergy, wheeze, current use of asthma medication, ever having asthma (significant as a potential predictor of asthma remission in adulthood) and self-reported allergic rhinitis. The derived model had an AUC of 0.75, but sensitivity and specificity values were not reported in the evaluation. The study sample and the survey used, however, limit its generalizability to other populations. The ISAAC survey used in the study has been previously validated only in children (modified versions of

ISAAC are available for adults but were not used by Deng et al.) and their sample consisted of only women aged 40 to 69 years.

A recent asthma screening tool was created by Sà-Sousa et al. to validate two screening tools for identifying asthmatic patients in surveys and clinical settings.[128] The authors used data from the Control and Burden of Asthma and Rhinitis (ICAR) cross-sectional study. The authors created two different scoring systems: the Adult Asthma Epidemiological Score (A2) derived from a literature review and the Global Allergy and Asthma Network of Excellence Score (GA2LEN) derived from the Global Allergy and Asthma Network of Excellence Survey study.

The difference between the two questionnaires is the A2 contains additional questions related to a previous history of a physician diagnosis whereas GA2LEN does not. At a score above 4, the validation cohort showed a 99.2% specificity for both scores, but low sensitivities of 48.3% for A2 and 37.9% for GA2LEN. The PPV was 93.3% (65.7-99.0) for A2 and 91.7% (59.7-98.8) for GA2LEN. However, the PPV needs to be interpreted with caution as the prevalence of asthma was almost 25% in the derivation and validation cohorts, a rate three times higher than the published prevalence of diagnosed cases in Canada and the USA. The AUC of the weighted score was 0.913 for A2 and 0.905 for the GA2LEN. Although the authors set aside 20% of the data to validate the scores, the scores were not externally or prospectively validated in real-time with participants, which is a significant limiting factor. Also, while the study objective was to design a screening tool to identify patients for a diagnosis work-up, another limiting factor was that four of the ten questions are related to whether the person currently has (or ever had) a physician diagnosis of asthma, been hospitalized for asthma, or currently has asthma attacks. Since the scoring was based on the sum of positive answers to the predictors in the multivariate logistic regression model, if a person had more positive (i.e., yes) answers, this resulted in a higher score. Thus, for individuals who do not have a diagnosis, or are unaware of their symptoms, may not meet the screening threshold and remain undiagnosed.

1.8   Rationale for book and Study Objectives

While spirometry is a valuable tool to identify OLD, the unavailability and inaccessibility of spirometry are significant barriers. These barriers have been attributed to financial costs and limited delivery of spirometry equipment to rural practices.[84,85] Identifying and managing OLD is critical to prevent adverse health outcomes and slow disease progression. This book project aims to develop a short, practical questionnaire to effectively identify persons with undiagnosed OLD. This book is significant considering the recent findings from the UCAP study. In a preliminary analysis, the UCAP study found that 20% of the initial 910 participants randomly recruited from across Canada, had reported respiratory symptoms, had no previous diagnosed lung disease, but did have OLD, as confirmed with lung function testing.[129] Moreover, the preliminary findings from UCAP had shown a low predictive ability for existing case-finding tools to accurately detect undiagnosed lung disease.

The book research objectives are:
1) To develop a questionnaire as an integral part of a case-finding strategy to identify undiagnosed COPD and asthma in symptomatic community-dwelling adults, and
2) To prospectively evaluate the ability of the developed questionnaire to accurately identify participants with undiagnosed COPD and asthma in the community

Thus, two distinct phases of the research will be involved:
1) A questionnaire derivation phase which addresses the first research objective
2) A questionnaire validation phase which addresses the second research objective

2. Methods

2.1 Study Design

This prospective, multi-site cohort study uses data collected between 19 June 2017 and 04 March 2020 from the Undiagnosed Chronic Obstructive Pulmonary Disease and Asthma Population (UCAP) cross-sectional study. The aim is to develop and validate a case-finding questionnaire to detect undiagnosed OLD. Sixteen study sites are participating in UCAP. Sites are located in Ottawa, Halifax, Montreal, Québec, Toronto x2, Barrie, Hamilton, Winnipeg, Calgary, Edmonton, Vancouver, Kingston, St. John's, London, and Saskatoon.

2.2 Inclusion and Exclusion Criteria

The inclusion and exclusion criteria, and study design for UCAP have been previously published.[128] Participants were recruited through random digit dialing to cellphones and landlines inside a 90-minute radius of the study sites. Participants were included in the study if, 1) informed consent was provided, 2) $\geq$18 years of age, and 3) experienced one or more respiratory symptoms (i.e., shortness of breath, wheezing, increased mucus or sputum, prolonged cough) in the past six months. All participants were screened for eligibility using the Asthma Screening Questionnaire (ASQ) regardless of age. Participants $\geq$60 years, and participants <60 years with a score of <6 on the ASQ, completed the Chronic Obstructive Pulmonary Disease Questionnaire (COPD-DQ). Participants scoring $\geq$19.5 points on the COPD-DQ or $\geq$6 on the ASQ were asked to complete a spirometry test at their local study site for confirmation of OLD.

2.3 Diagnosis of Obstructive Lung Disease

At the study site, a diagnosis of OLD was assessed using spirometry. Lung testing was done by certified study personnel. Participants were diagnosed with asthma if FEV_1 improved by $\geq$12% and $\geq$200 mL following bronchodilator administration of 400ug of salbutamol. Participants were diagnosed with COPD if the post-bronchodilation FEV_1/FVC ratio was below the lower limit of the 95% confidence interval for healthy participants of identical sex, age and height.

2.4 Data extraction

The pool of potential questions used to develop the case-finding questionnaire to detect undiagnosed OLD was selected from the questionnaires listed below. Study participants completed the ASQ at eligibility screening and the other five questionnaires during their spirometry visit. The text of each individual questionnaire can be found in **Appendix A.**

1. COPD Assessment Test (CAT)
2. Short Form-36 Quality of Life Questionnaire (SF-36 QoL)
3. Work, Productivity and Impairment: General Health (WPAIGH) Questionnaire
4. The St. George's Respiratory Questionnaire (SGRQ)
5. Asthma Screening Questionnaire (ASQ)
6. COPD Diagnostic Questionnaire (COPD-DQ)
7. Personal Information Sheet

Other than the Personal Information Sheet, all the questionnaires, including the ASQ, have been previously published.[118,126,130] All but ASQ have been validated with selected populations but none has been validated for a population of symptomatic adults with undiagnosed respiratory disease. The Personal Information Sheet refers to a study-specific data collection form with questions related to occupational and medical history, smoking exposures (including marijuana exposure, pet exposure) and access to healthcare services. Since participants meeting a score ≥ 6 for the ASQ were already deemed eligible to undergo spirometry, the COPD-DQ was only administered to 637 of the 1615 participants (39%) and was, thus, excluded from the potential pool of candidate predictor questions.

The SF-36 QoL and WPAIGH were not questionnaires designed to predict undiagnosed chronic respiratory diseases. Many of the questions in the SF-36 QoL, however, contain predictors or risk factors related to obstructive lung disease, such as physical activity limitations and mental well-being.[102,131] Similarly the WPAIGH contains potentially relevant questions related to loss of days at work due to illness.[61]

2.5 Outcome Measure

Based on the spirometry results, participants were categorized into three mutually exclusive diagnostic groups: no OLD, asthma alone, and COPD. Participants satisfying spirometry criteria for both asthma and COPD were classified in the COPD outcome category. Both asthma and COPD fall under the classification of obstructive lung diseases and while the outcome could be a binary classification of no OLD versus OLD, a three-level outcome was better suited to differentiate and identify disease-specific risk factors.

2.6 Model Development

The primary objective of the book was to develop a case-finding questionnaire effective in detecting undiagnosed OLD in symptomatic community-dwelling adults. Two modeling techniques were used to build a final model strongly predictive of undiagnosed OLD: 1) a multinomial logistic regression using backward elimination, and 2) recursive partitioning using the classification and regression trees (CART) method. Developed by Leo Breiman et al., CART does not require assumptions about the data distribution, can handle missing values, requires no transformations of the data, identifies higher order interactions, and is presented as a hierarchical diagram.[132,133] Findings from different modeling algorithms were compared to develop a robust prediction model.

With backward elimination, the model first begins with inclusion of all the candidate predictors. During the process, predictors with a p-value greater than a predetermined threshold are eliminated. This process is repeated until all predictors remaining in the model have a significance level below the threshold for either one or both diseases. Default parameters were set for backward elimination in STATA for a multinomial logistic regression model. A p-value of 0.05 was set as the threshold for removal.

In comparison, CART is a non-parametric, statistical modeling technique where a tree is created through a binary recursive partitioning algorithm. At each node, CART selects the best predictor variable and splitting criterion (i.e., cut-off value) to create subgroups with similar values of the outcome.[134]

The following section describes the model development, first consisting of data preparation specific to each modeling algorithm and purposeful selection of candidate predictors to be used for both methods and followed by a comparative evaluation of their predictive performance. The final model selected will be subsequently referred to as the UCAP Questionnaire.

2.6.1   Choosing the Candidate Pool of Predictor Variables

The candidate pool of predictors (to be used for multinomial logistic regression and CART) consisted of variables constructed from the questions of the CAT, SF-36 QoL, SGRQ, WPAIGH, ASQ, and Personal Information Sheet. The suitability of the predictors to be included in the candidate pool involved comprehensive literature review, clinical judgment, and the statistical association between each potential predictor and the outcome. A univariate analysis was conducted to evaluate the strength of association between the outcome and predictor. The associations of categorical variables were assessed using a $\mathcal{X}^2$ test of independence and continuous measures were assessed using ANOVA, or a Kruskal-Wallis test of independence if data were skewed. Variables significant at a p-value of <0.25 and deemed clinically relevant were added to the candidate pool of predictors for regression. A p-value below <0.20 to 0.25 has been a recommended threshold for initial variable screening as opposed to a p-value less than 0.05 for model building.[135,136] This threshold is distinct from the usual 0.05 value that is used in practice for statistical significance. While this high p-value threshold may admit some variables of questionable importance, it avoids losing potentially valuable predictors from the model development pool as the variables can become significant when combined with other predictors.[135]

2.6.1.1 Collinearity and Missing Data

Given the questionnaires had questions that were nearly identical, collinearity of variables was assessed to remove related variables. Alongside a manual assessment of collinearity, the backward elimination process in STATA automatically removes similar variables that either add little or no predictive power to the model. Other measures for collinearity assessment are available. For this book, a variable was omitted if the variance inflation factor was greater than 2.5 when included with another variable or multiple variables, depending on the number of collinear variables. There is evidence of multicollinearity when a variable is insignificant in a multivariate regression yet is significant in a univariate regression model, or vice versa. To uncover significant changes in beta-coefficients or p-values, or any inflation of standard errors, similar variables were first examined by univariate regression, and then combined in a multivariate regression model.

The overall rate of missing values for predictors in the candidate pool ranged from 0% to 2.6%, with one variable at 5.5% missing. The following conditional question in the SGRQ, "Questions about your medication:" and "If taking no medication go straight go to Section 6.", was omitted from the candidate pool because 70% of the responses were missing as valid skips. When the valid skip responses were coded as an indicator variable, it was found not predictive of undiagnosed OLD based on univariate association. A cross-tabulation also showed a relatively small count of outcome events (<10) for each OLD. Indicator variables (i.e., 'unknown' category) were created for missing values for some questions, such as the question about primary or second-hand smoke exposure, wheezing during the morning, and ASQ questions as a pattern of missingness was observed.

2.6.2 Multinomial Logistic Regression
2.6.2.1 Transformation of Ordinal Variables

Prior to doing so, the ordinal variables from the CAT and the SF-36 QoL questionnaires were transformed using fitted logistic regression functions. Based on the relationships observed between item responses and outcomes of each disease, the original questions, although having scales that were structured as ordinal, demonstrated non-monotonic associations between the outcome risk and rating responses. This characteristic was found by Preteroti et al. and therefore similarly addressed here using fitted logistic regression transformations.[129]

To illustrate the transformation for the CAT item "I never cough" to "I cough all the time," the scale ranges from 0 to 6. Coughing is a known symptom of OLD, but the frequency distribution of the outcome does not show a monotonic association with the rating. Based on a tabulation of the cough rating against the multi-leveled outcome, the frequency of cases for each disease increased until a score of 3, where the frequency peaked, and afterwards decreased.

A multinomial logistic regression was used to model the relation of the disease outcome to the responses for ordinal-scaled questions. The risk score for each participant, calculated from the fitted logistic model, is the estimated log-odds for the disease outcome based on the participant's response to the question. The six unique risk scores generated for the cough variable in relation to the outcome of COPD are shown in **Table 2.**

Table 2. Example of logistic response scores for the 'cough' CAT question for the outcome of COPD

CAT Response for Cough	Logistic Score for Cough
0	-1.273
1	-2.120
2	-2.464
3	-2.326
4	-2.132
5	-2.236

2.6.2.2 Implementing Question Selection Using Multinomial Logistic Regression

To build the logistic regression model, the candidate pool of predictors was entered into a backward elimination procedure for the 'mlogit' function in STATA. The questions that were not eliminated by the procedure constitute the UCAP Questionnaire selected by this method.

2.6.3   Recursive Partitioning: Classification and Regression Trees

To build the decision tree, the dataset was randomly split into a derivation sample (80%) and validation sample (20%) in which the model was developed using the derivation sample and then evaluated on the validation sample. General recommendations have been to use 60% to 80% for training the data with the remaining 40% to 20% for testing the model. The 80:20 split has been recommended as a start point, and this ratio was found to be suitable to build the tree.[137]

The decision tree was developed with the 'rpart' (R Studio Software Version 1.4.1103) package to support the multi-class outcome. The same candidate pool of predictors used in the logistic regression model-building was used for the CART method.

A descriptive comparison of demographic and clinical characteristics of the derivation sample (N=1293) and validation sample (N=322) is shown in the Results section. The split-train validation method was selected to validate the model since the 'rpart' package, by default, applies 10-fold cross-validation to minimize the prediction error with changing tree size.[138] Random partitioning is expected to produce matching distributions of the data, however, randomly sub-splitting the original dataset through train-split validation can potentially skew the distribution of the characteristics and outcome.[139] **Table 9** was used to illustrate the similar characteristics of both samples, as anticipated. For the model, no specific splits were forced into the tree and no pruning was performed for the tree.

2.6.4   Predictive Performance

Predictive performance of each model was characterized by its discrimination and calibration. The performance of the models was assessed and compared using the area under the receiver operating characteristic curve for discrimination, abbreviated AUC and ROC respectively. Predictive performance of the model was considered acceptable if the AUC was between 0.70 and 0.80, and considered to have no discrimination if the AUC was 0.50 or less.[140] The calibration of the logistic regression model was assessed using a version of the Hosmer-

Lemeshow goodness-of-fit test for a multinomial logistic regression, created by Hosmer and W. Fagerland ('mlogitgof') in STATA 16.1.[141]

Internal validation using k-fold cross-validation was used to assess overfitting of the regression model and predictive ability. Using k-fold cross validation, the sample is partitioned into k equal-sized subsamples, or folds. A single fold is used for validation while the other k-1 folds are used for training the model.[142] The procedure is repeated k times until each fold has been used to test the model. Repeated cross-fold validation is the same, but repeated n times. Other robust forms of internal validation are available, such as bootstrapping. Cross-validation was selected based on familiarity of the validation method.

With the final selected model, a risk cut-off for the outcome prediction was determined by assessing the sensitivity and specificity at different thresholds.

2.7 Face Validity and Readability

The UCAP Questionnaire was to be evaluated using an acceptability and face validity survey (**Appendix B**). The survey was provided to a sample of clinicians at The Ottawa Hospital via email and a sample of participants from the UCAP study via telephone. The reading level of the UCAP Questionnaire was also assessed using the Flesch-Kincaid Reading Ease and Flesch-Kincaid Grade Level. Reading Ease is evaluated based on the average number of syllables per word and the average sentence length. The Flesch-Kincaid Reading Ease is scored from 0 to 100, with scores above 70 indicating easy readability.[143] The Flesch-Kincaid Grade Level indicates the grade level in the American school system necessary to comprehend the text of the questionnaire. The feedback would provide insight into the clarity of the questions, suitability of the wording and order of presentation. The readability of the UCAP Questionnaire was assessed using Microsoft Word Version 16.30.

2.8 Reliability

The reliability of the UCAP Questionnaire was assessed using a test-retest comparison to determine whether the participants' responses remained similar on two different occasions. Participants were contacted by telephone to complete the questionnaire at two time points one week apart. Common time intervals for test-retest are between one to two weeks. The interval was set long enough so participants cannot reproduce their previous responses by simple recall, but short enough that they may not experience real health changes in the interim between the first and second time points.[144,145]

To assess the reliability of the questions, the intraclass correlation coefficient (ICC; two-way mixed effects model) was used for continuous variables. Different measures of reliability (e.g., Pearson correlation coefficient, t-test) are available; however, the ICC is the most preferable and frequently used measure. Quadratic weighted Kappa was used to assess the ordinal variables and unweighted Kappa for the categorical variables. Due to the ranking of ordinal data, a weighing scheme accounts for the magnitude of differences between the categories where more weight is applied when disagreements, or differences, between the two ratings are greater in scale.[146] Stratification of the results by age was used to determine whether results varied by different groups.

Bland-Altman plots were combined with the ICC for the continuous variables. The Bland-Altman is a plot of the average of the two measurements (time 1 and time 2) against the differences in the measurements.[147] With the plot, a visual interpretation of the systematic differences, the range of values, and the variation of the results using the limits of agreement, can be assessed. The limits of agreement are calculated by the mean difference ± 1.96 standard deviations; and as a general recommendation, approximately 95% of the mean differences should lie between the limits.

The ICC was interpreted as: less than 0.50, poor; 0.50 to 0.75, moderate; 0.75 to 0.90, good; and above 0.90, excellent.[148] Kappa was interpreted as: <0.2, slight; 0.21-0.40, fair; 0.41-0.60, moderate; 0.61-0.80, substantial; and 0.81-1.00, almost perfect.[148,149]

2.9 External Validation

To prospectively validate the risk score of the UCAP Questionnaire, a new cohort of participants was recruited from the UCAP study between October 2020 and January 2021 at study sites open during the COVID-19 pandemic. Inclusion criteria were modified to incorporate the new questionnaire: participants were eligible to enter the UCAP study and proceed to spirometry if they had a score of ≥ 6 on the ASQ, a score of ≥ 20 on the COPD-DQ, or a risk score (probability) of $\geq 6\%$ for either asthma or COPD on the UCAP Questionnaire

2.9.1   Sample Size

The desired sample size for external validation was determined for each disease using the AUC as the performance measure of interest. Based on previous findings from the UCAP study,[129] the estimated prevalence for undiagnosed COPD and undiagnosed asthma was 12% and 8% respectively. For COPD, a sample of 452 participants achieves a two-sided 95% confidence interval with a 0.2 precision for a target AUC of 0.85. For asthma, a sample of 313 participants achieves the same precision for a target AUC of 0.75. As a result, a minimum sample size of 497 participants (accounting for 10% dropout) would estimate an AUC of 0.75 for asthma and an AUC of 0.85 for COPD with a precision of at least 0.20.

However, this desired sample size for the prospective validation phase could not be achieved during the expected timeframe because of COVID-related study site closures with consequent significant slowing of recruitment into the UCAP study. As a result, the number of participants recruited for test-retest and external validation are lower than planned. The analyses, however, were still conducted to provide a pilot view of the findings.

2.10   Ethics Board Approval

Clinical Trials Ontario (CTO) and the Research Ethics Board (CTO) representing the 16 participating UCAP study sites reviewed and approved the amendment of the test-retest reliability and external validation participation forms and consented to the extended UCAP protocol prior to initiating the study (**Appendix C**).

2.11 Statistical Software

Statistical analyses were performed using STATA (StataCorp, College Station, TX, USA) Version 16.1 and R Studio Software, Version 1.4.1103.

3. Results

3.1 Study Sample for the Derivation Phase of the UCAP Questionnaire

Figure 1 illustrates a flow diagram of the enrolled participants. 1702 participants were enrolled between June 2017 and March 2020 into the UCAP study from 16 study sites. Among these participants, 50 were randomly selected and reserved for hold-out for the validation phase in case the UCAP study was forced to remain closed during the COVID-19 pandemic and new participants for the validation exercise would therefore not be available. These 50 subjects were ultimately not analyzed for purposes of this book. From the remaining 1652 participants, 37 were omitted due to inadequate spirometry. A total of 1615 participants were included in the questionnaire derivation phase of the study, of which 195 participants (12%) were diagnosed with COPD and 136 participants (8%) were diagnosed with asthma based on the spirometric diagnostic criteria outlined earlier.

Figure 1. Flowchart of enrolled UCAP participants.

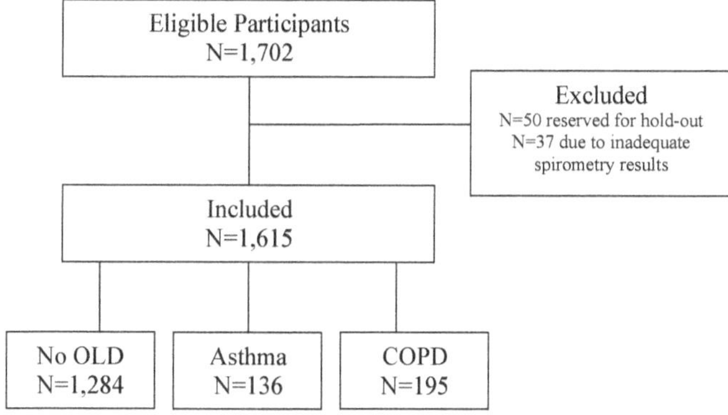

3.2 Multinomial Logistic Regression Model

Table 3. Demographic and clinical characteristics according to diagnosis of OLD (N=1,615)

Characteristics	No obstructive lung disease (OLD) N=1284	Asthma N=136	COPD N=195
Age, year[†]	61 (48-70)	60 (48-71)	67 (59-74)
Sex (n, %)			
Female	654 (51)	58 (43)	70 (36)
Male	630 (49)	78 (57)	125 (64)
Race/Ethnicity (n, %)			
Caucasian	1,178 (92)	127 (93)	188 (97)
Asian	56 (4)	5 (4)	1 (0.5)
American Indian, Alaska Native, Native Hawaiian, Hispanic or Latino, Mixed	24 (2)	2 (1.5)	4 (2)
Black or African American	26 (2)	2 (1.5)	1 (0.5)
Level of education (n, %)			
High school or less	359 (28)	42 (31)	75 (38)
Some college/university	174 (14)	21 (15)	24 (12)
College/university	712 (55)	71 (52)	87 (45)
Prefers not to answer	39 (3)	2 (2)	9 (5)
Smoking history (n, %)			
Current	223 (17)	20 (15)	84 (43)
Former	508 (40)	61 (45)	86 (44)
Never	533 (43)	55 (40)	25 (13)
Comorbidities (n, %)[†]			
GERD	473 (37)	48 (36)	64 (34)
Stroke	53 (4)	1 (1)	8 (4)
Coronary artery disease	108 (8)	10 (8)	39 (20)
Hypertension	447 (35)	42 (31)	70 (37)
Depression/Anxiety	492 (39)	52 (39)	64 (34)
Diabetes mellitus	176 (14)	16 (12)	28 (15)
Occupational exposure (n, %)			
Yes	488 (38)	58 (44)	95 (49)
No	792 (62)	75 (56)	100 (51)
Pre-bronchodilator spirometry[†]			
FEV_1	2.78 (2.21-3.36)	2.45 (1.90-3.06)	1.98 (1.44-2.42)
FEV_1 % predicted	96 (86-106)	82 (74-91)	71 (59-82)
FEV_1/FVC	77 (73-80)	69 (64-74)	60 (54-64)
Post-bronchodilator spirometry[†]			
FEV_1	2.86 (2.28-3.47)	2.80 (2.21-3.49)	2.09 (1.57-2.62)
FEV_1 % predicted	99 (89-109)	95 (87-103)	76 (65-86)
FEV_1/FVC	79 (75-83)	75 (70-80)	62 (57-66)

Abbreviations: FEV_1=forced expiratory volume in a second; FVC=forced vital capacity; GERD=gastroesophageal reflux disease. [†] Data are presented as median (P25-P75)

Table 3 summarizes the clinical and demographic characteristics of the UCAP sample. The median age was 60 years for the asthma group and 67 years for the COPD group; over 50% of the COPD and asthma groups were male. The smoking histories of no OLD and asthma subjects are similar but differ sharply from COPD subjects who are more often current smokers than never smokers. Similar prevalence rates of comorbidities were found in all three diagnosis groups, other than history of coronary artery disease (20% in the COPD group versus 8% in the other groups).

Each of the potential predictors for model development was investigated for its univariate association with the disease outcome. The predictor list and their associated levels of significance are presented in **Appendix D**.

While STATA does implement automatic elimination of collinear predictors in the stepwise 'mlogit' function, a manual review for collinearity was conducted. In particular, a group of questions related to walking included, 1) *Walking more than one kilometer*, 2) *Walking several hundred meters*, 3) *Walking one hundred meters*, 4) *I walk slower than other people, or I stop for rests*, 5) *If I hurry or walk fast, I have to stop or slow down*, and 6) *Walking outside on the level*. Another set of questions related to climbing hills or stairs included, 1) *Climbing up a flight of stairs*, 2) *Climbing hills*, 3) *When I walk up a hill or one flight of stairs I am not breathless* to *When I walk up a hill or one flight of stairs I am very breathless*, 4) *Climbing several flights of stairs*, 5) *Climbing one flight of stairs*, and 6) *If I climb up one flight of stairs, I have to go slow or stop*. Other questions related to physical activity: 1) *Vigorous activities*, 2) *Limited in moderate activities*, 3) *My breathing makes it difficult to do things such as climbing up hills, carrying things upstairs, light gardening such as weeding, dancing, bowling or golfing*, 4) *My breathing makes it difficult to do things such as carrying heavy loads, digging the garden or shovelling snow, jogging or walking at 5 kilometers per hour, playing tennis or swimming*, and 5) *My breathing makes it difficult to do things such as very heavy manual work, running, cycling, swimming fast or playing competitive sports*. Only one of the questions in a similar group was arbitrarily retained as a potential predictor.

The final pool of variables selected from each questionnaire were the following:

Demographic and Clinical Variables: Age, Sex, Pack-years of cigarette smoking, Exposure to primary or second-hand smoke, $\geq$3 Months of sandblasting or paint exposure, Hospitalization for breathing problems or respiratory illness, Smoke marijuana, Use of Salbutamol (Ventolin)

CAT: Cough, Phlegm, Chest tightness, Sleep, Lung

SF-36 QoL: Limited in vigorous activities, Limited walking more than one kilometer, Cut down on amount of time spent on work/activities as a result of emotional problems, Feeling tired during past four weeks, Feeling worn out during past four weeks, I seem to get sick a little easier than other people

SGRQ: Shortness of breath in the past three months, Number of severe attacks of chest problems, Worsening of wheeze in morning, Sitting or lying still, Painful cough, Breathless when bending over, I feel I am not in control of my chest problem, I take long time to get washed or dressed, If I climb up stairs I have to go slowly, If I hurry or walk fast, I have to stop or slow down

WPAI-GH: Hours missed from work due to breathing problems in past seven days

ASQ: Worsening of cough, chest tightness, or wheeze when lying down to sleep, Worsening of shortness of breath, wheeze, chest after exercise, Worsening of chest tightness, wheeze after laughing or crying

Tables 4 and **5** show the final multinomial logistic regression model. The resultant model consisted of 13 predictors: age, pack-years of cigarette smoking, primary or second-hand smoking exposure, $\geq$3 months of exposure to sandblasting and/or paint, use of salbutamol medication, wheezing during the morning, frequency of chest problems, cough, chest tightness, sleep, physical activity limitations, tiredness, and emotional health.

The ASQ variable derived from the question, "Worsening of coughing after laughing or crying" was initially selected based on its statistical predictive contribution but upon consultation was found to lack clinical validity and therefore removed. Contrary to clinical experience, the direction of association was negative for both asthma and COPD indicating that the risk of either lung disease would decrease if the response was yes. The variable was not found to be collinear with other questions. Univariate and multivariate regression models still showed the same negative direction of association. A comparison of the regression coefficients in a multinomial logistic model with and without the variable showed changes in the coefficients were less than 10%.[150]

Overall, six predictors were found to be significant for asthma: occupational exposure to paint, chemical, fumes, and sandblasting, wheezing during the morning, frequency of severe chest problems, cough, chest tightness, and emotional health. Nine predictors were found to be significant for COPD: age, pack-years of cigarette smoke, primary or second-hand smoke exposure, salbutamol medication, wheezing during the morning, sleep, chest tightness, physical activity limitation, and tiredness. The two predictors, 'Wheeze during the morning' and 'Chest tightness' are the only questions among the 13 that were significant for both asthma and COPD, with wheezing having almost identical logistic regression coefficients for each disease.

3.2.1   Modification to the Original Model

To derive the final model, a modification was made to improve the clinical validity. Prior to implementing the case-finding UCAP Questionnaire, the predicted probabilities of risk were assessed. As a result of the underlying data distribution of the sample, a score of "0" on the "Cough" question significantly inflated the probability of disease. In addition, other assessments of the unadjusted logistic regression model with only "Cough," found a score of "0" had the highest risk of asthma compared to all the other categories. To remedy this aberration, the categories of 0 and 1 were combined into one category, resulting in the updated model presented below. No significant inflation of the risk probability was found after this modification. The original thresholds selected for the risk scores were retained for the modified model.

Table 4. Risk Scoring for Asthma based on the Multinomial Logistic Regression Model

Question [Scale]	β-coefficient	95% CI	p-value[*]
1. How old are you? [years]	-0.0040	-0.017-0.009	0.554
2. Are you currently smoking cigarettes or have you smoked cigarettes in the past? **If yes**, please indicate the number of years you have spent smoking and the average number of cigarette packs per day (20 cigarettes = 1.0 pack) [pack-years]	0.0021	-0.010-0.014	0.728
3. Are you regularly exposed to cigarette smoke (either from yourself, or from people around you) on a daily basis? [Yes/No]	-0.3929	-0.892-0.106	0.123
4. a. Have you ever worked for <u>3 months or more</u> with paint, chemicals, or fumes? **If yes**, how many months did you work? [months] b. Have you ever worked for <u>3 months or more</u> with sandblasting? **If yes**, how many months did you work? [months]	0.9402	0.337-1.54	**0.002**
5. Are you currently taking the medication Salbutamol (also known as Ventolin) for your breathing? [Yes/No]	0.4124	-0.097-0.922	0.112
6. If you have a wheeze, is it worse in the morning? [Not Applicable/Yes/No]	0.5799	0.183-0.977	**0.004**
7. During the past 3 months, how many severe or very unpleasant attacks of chest problems (attacks of shortness of breath or wheezing) have you had? [More than 3 attacks/3 attacks/2 attacks/1 attack/No attack]	0.8850	0.241-1.529	**0.007**
8. Please rate your <u>cough</u> on a scale of 0 to 5 with 0 meaning I never cough to 5 meaning I cough all the time.	1.4153	0.271-2.56	**0.015**

Question [Scale]	β-coefficient	95% CI	p-value[*]
9. Please rate your <u>sleep</u> on a scale of 0 to 5 with 0 meaning I sleep soundly to 5 meaning I do not sleep soundly because of my lung condition.	0.3983	-0.627-1.424	0.446
10. Please rate your <u>chest tightness</u> on a scale of 0 to 5 with 0 meaning no chest tightness at all to 5 meaning my chest feels very tight.	0.9034	0.242-1.57	**0.007**
11. Does your health <u>now</u> limit you in vigorous activities, such as running, lifting heavy objects, or participating in strenuous sports? [Yes, limited a lot/Yes, limited a little/No, not limited at all]	0.0876	-0.367-0.542	0.706
12. How much of the time during the past 4 weeks, did you feel tired? [All of the time/Most of the time/Some of the time/A little of the time/None]	-0.2503	-0.918-0.417	0.462
13. During the past 4 weeks, how much of the time have you had to cut down on the amount of time you spent on work or other regular activities as a result of any emotional problems, such as feeling depressed or anxious? [All of the time/Most of the time/Some of the time/A little of the time/None]	1.0199	0.273-1.77	**0.007**
Constant	9.8758		

Table 5. Risk Scoring for COPD based on the Multinomial Logistic Regression Model

Question [Scale]	β-coefficient	95% CI	p-value[*]
1. How old are you? [years]	0.0421	0.026-0.059	**0.000**
2. Are you currently smoking cigarettes or have you smoked cigarettes in the past? **If yes**, please indicate the number of years you have spent smoking and the average number of cigarette packs per day (20 cigarettes = 1.0 pack) [pack-years]	0.0307	0.023-0.039	**0.000**
3. Are you regularly exposed to cigarette smoke (either from yourself, or from people around you) on a daily basis? [Yes/No]	1.2308	0.826-1.64	**0.000**

Question			
4. a. Have you ever worked for <u>3 months or more</u> with paint, chemicals, or fumes? **If yes**, how many months did you work? [months]	0.0248	-0.919-0.969	0.959
b. Have you ever worked for <u>3 months or more</u> with sandblasting? **If yes**, how many months did you work? [months]			
5. Are you currently taking the medication Salbutamol (also known as Ventolin) for your breathing? [Yes/No]	0.8222	0.339-1.31	**0.001**
6. If you have a wheeze, is it worse in the morning? [Not Applicable/Yes/No]	0.5766	0.196-0.956	**0.003**
7. During the past 3 months, how many severe or very unpleasant attacks of chest problems (attacks of shortness of breath or wheezing) have you had? [3 attacks and more/3 attacks/2 attacks/1 attack/No attack]	-0.1762	-0.874-0.522	0.621
8. Please rate your <u>cough</u> on a scale of 0 to 5 with 0 meaning I never cough to 5 meaning I cough all the time.	0.8339	-0.205-1.87	0.116
9. Please rate your <u>sleep</u> on a scale of 0 to 5 with 0 meaning I sleep soundly to 5 meaning I do not sleep soundly because of my lung condition.	1.3127	0.291-2.33	**0.012**
10. Please rate your <u>chest tightness</u> on a scale of 0 to 5 with 0 meaning no chest tightness at all to 5 meaning my chest feels very tight.	-0.1418	0.242-1.57	**0.007**
11. Does your health <u>now</u> limit you in vigorous activities, such as running, lifting heavy objects, or participating in strenuous sports? [Yes, limited a lot/Yes, limited a little/No, not limited at all]	0.9059	0.416-1.40	**0.000**
12. How much of the time during the past 4 weeks, did you feel tired? [All of the time/Most of the time/Some of the time/A little of the time/None]	1.1414	0.441-1.84	**0.001**

13. During the past 4 weeks, how much of the time have you had to cut down on the amount of time you spent on work or other regular activities as a result of any emotional problems, such as feeling depressed or anxious? [All of the time/Most of the time/Some of the time/A little of the time/None]	0.0105	-0.548-0.569	0.971
Constant	1.6776		

3.2.2   Risk Score and Cut-Offs

The risk scores for asthma and COPD were the predicted probabilities calculated from the following regression equations:

$$\Pr(Y_1 = COPD) = \frac{exp\,[X1]}{1 + exp[X1] + exp\,[X2]} \quad \text{and} \quad \Pr(Y_2 = Asthma) = \frac{exp\,[X2]}{1 + exp[X1] + exp\,[X2]}$$

where X1 is equal to (0.0421xAge) + (0.0307xPack-Years) + (1.2308xSmoke Exposure) + [(0.0248)x(-2.274+(Paint x-0.0005) + (Sandx0.0061))] + (0.8222xVentolin) + (0.5766xWheeze) + (-0.1762xChest problems) + (0.8339xCough) + (1.3127xSleep) + (-0.1418xChest tightness) + (0.9059xActivities) + (1.1414xTired) + (0.0105xEmotional health) + 1.6776, and, where X2 is equal to (0.0040xAge) + (0.0021xPack-Years) + (-0.3929xSmoke Exposure) + [(0.9402)x(-2.274+(Paint x -0.0005) + (Sandx0.0061))] + (0.4124xVentolin) + (0.5799xWheeze) + (0.8850xChest problems) + (1.4153xCough) + (0.3983xSleep) + (0.9034xChest tightness) + (0.0876xActivities) + (-0.2503xTired) + (1.0199xEmotional health) + 9.8758.

The same method applied to the ordinal questions in Section 2.6.2.1 was applied to the occupational exposure variable, "Have you ever worked for 3 months or more with…" to combine two significant predictors of OLD: 1) sandblasting exposure, and 2) paint, chemicals, and fume exposure. The risk score generated was based on the multinomial logistic equation for the asthma outcome: (-2.274(constant)+(Months of Paint x-0.0005) + (Months of Sandx0.0061)). The UCAP Questionnaire (web-calculator displayed in **Figure 2**) can be accessed online through the following link: https://omc.ohri.ca/UCAPquestionnaire/.

Figure 2. The online calculator for the UCAP Questionnaire.

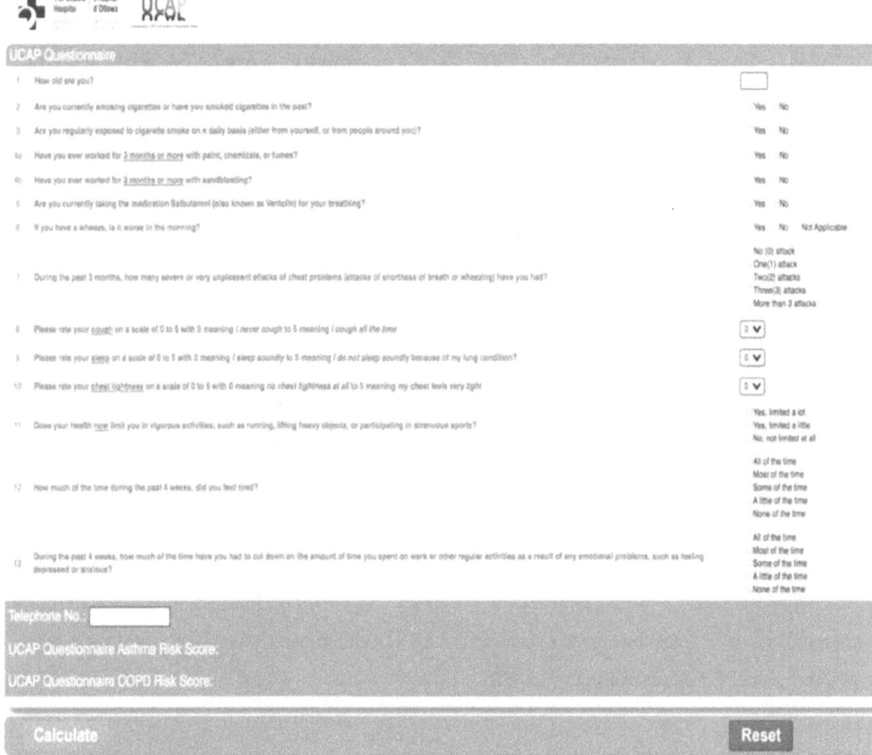

To determine the best risk cut-offs for asthma and COPD, the sensitivity, specificity, positive predictive values and negative predictive values of different cut-offs (**Table 6**) were calculated for each disease.

Table 6. Associated sensitivity, specificity, PPV, and NPV values (%) at varying cut-offs for each disease

Risk Cut-Off (%)	Asthma				COPD			
	Sensitivity	Specificity	PPV	NPV	Sensitivity	Specificity	PPV	NPV
5	87	37	11	96	91	47	19	97
10	54	74	16	94	78	70	25	96
15	36	89	21	93	65	82	33	95
20	18	96	28	92	56	88	41	94

A 2x3 classification table was constructed using STATA to apply specific opportunity costs to determine the most appropriate cut-off for each disease. Cost-classification matrices can be used when costs of false negatives and false positives are different in order to minimize the total incurred cost of prediction errors. For the cost matrix adopted in this application, a false negative for asthma was assigned a higher cost than was assigned for COPD. The reasons being, asthma tends to afflict younger persons compared to COPD, the risk of morbidity associated with asthma is significant, and, effective therapies are available for successful management of asthma. Based on clinical judgment, we assigned an incurred cost of 10 units for a false negative for asthma, an incurred cost of 8 units for a false negative for COPD, and an incurred cost of 1 unit for a false positive signal for either asthma or COPD.

Applying the assigned costs to the logistic regression model and using a cost-minimization strategy determined the most appropriate risk cut-off was greater than or equal to 6% for each disease. Based on **Table 7**, applying risk cut-offs of 6% for each disease to the derivation sample yielded a specificity of 17% for no-OLD, a sensitivity of 91% for asthma, and 96% sensitivity for COPD. **Table 8** displays the varying sensitivity, specificity, PPV, and NPV at different cut-offs using the specified costs.

Table 7. Classification table at a risk cut-off of $\geq 6\%$ against the true state of disease for asthma and COPD

Disease Prediction	True Disease			Total	PPV/NPV
	No OLD	**Asthma**	**COPD**		
Yes	1036 (FP)	123 (TP1)	183 (TP2)	1342	PPV 23%
No	219 (TN)	12 (FN1)	7 (FN2)	238	NPV 92%
Total	1255	135	190	N=1580	--
Sensitivity	--	91%	96%	--	--
Specificity	17%	--	--	--	--

PPV=Positive Predictive Value; NPV=Negative Predictive Value; FP=False Positive; TP=True Positive

Table 8. Associated sensitivity, specificity, PPV, and NPV values (%) at varying cut-offs for each disease

Risk Cut-Off (%)	Asthma Sensitivity	COPD Sensitivity	No OLD Specificity	PPV	NPV
5	97	99	10	22	95
6	91	96	17	23	92
10	64	82	47	27	88
15	38	70	72	34	86
20	24	61	85	44	85

3.2.3 UCAP Questionnaire Performance

The AUC was 0.69 (95% CI: 0.64-0.74) for asthma and 0.82 (95% CI: 0.78-0.86) for COPD
(**Figure 3**). The AUC of combining both disorders was 0.71 (95% CI: 0.68-0.75). The Hosmer-
Lemeshow goodness of fit statistic was 23.44 (16 degrees of freedom) with a corresponding p-
value of 0.102, indicating a reasonably fitted model. Internal validation of the model was
performed using repeated k-fold cross validation. The final model was cross-validated using a
10-fold method with 1000 repeated samples. The cross-validation produced average AUC values
of 0.64 (95% CI: 0.45-0.80) for asthma and 0.79 (95% CI: 0.70-0.90) for COPD.

Figure 3. Receiver operating characteristic curve for UCAP Questionnaire. AUC= 0.69 for
asthma, AUC= 0.82 for COPD, AUC= 0.71 for either asthma or COPD.

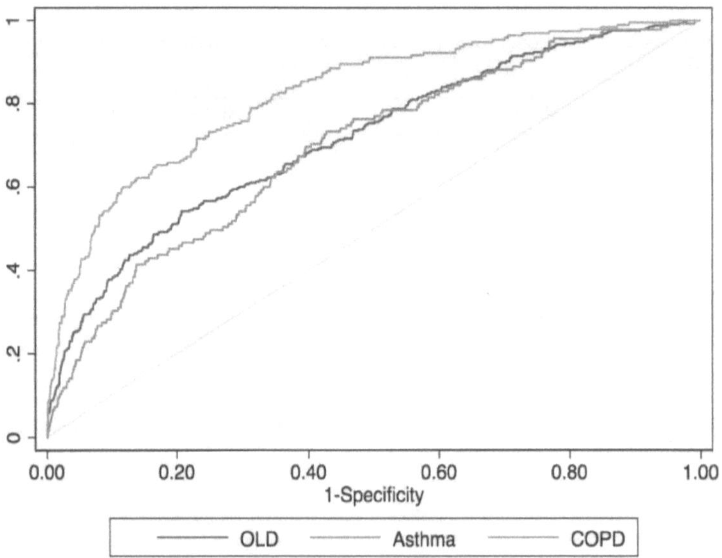

3.3 Recursive Partitioning: Classification and Regression Trees

From the 1615 participants, a random split of 1293 (80%) participants and 322 (20%)
participants was used to create respective derivation and internal validation samples.
Characteristics of the derivation and internal validation samples are shown in **Table 9**.

Table 9. Demographic and clinical characteristics of derivation and validation samples

Characteristics	Total N=1615	Derivation Sample N=1293	Validation Sample N=322
Age, year[†]	61 (21)	62 (21)	60 (19)
Sex (n, %)			
Female	782 (48)	618 (48)	164 (51)
Male	833 (52)	675 (52)	158 (49)
Smoking history (n, %)			
Current	327 (20)	258 (20)	69 (21)
Former	655 (41)	524 (41)	122 (38)
Never	633 (39)	511 (40)	131 (41)
Race/Ethnicity (n, %)			
Caucasian	1,493(92)	1194 (92)	299 (93)
Asian	62 (4)	40 (4)	12 (4)
American Indian, Alaska Native, Native Hawaiian, Hispanic or Latino, Mixed	31 (2)	23 (2)	4 (1)
Black or African American	29 (2)	23 (2)	6 (2)
Pre-bronchodilator spirometry[†]			
FEV_1	2.64 (1.17)	2.65 (1.15)	2.62 (1.23)
FEV_1 % predicted	92 (23)	92 (23)	94 (22)
FEV_1/FVC	75 (11)	75 (11)	76 (9)
Post-bronchodilator spirometry[†]			
FEV_1	2.77 (1.2)	2.78 (1.17)	2.73 (1.29)
FEV_1 % predicted	96 (21)	96 (22)	98 (21)
FEV_1/FVC	78 (10)	78 (10)	78 (10)
Presence of OLD (n, %)	331 (21)	262 (20)	66 (21)
Asthma (n, %)	136 (8)	109 (8)	27 (8)
COPD (n, %)	195 (27)	156 (12)	39 (12)

Abbreviations: FEV_1=forced expiratory volume in a second; FVC=forced vital capacity; OLD=obstructive
lung disease; COPD=chronic obstructive pulmonary disease [†]Data are presented as median (interquartile
range)

The resulting CART decision tree is shown in **Figure 4**; the decision tree identified the following four predictors as most efficient in classifying the diagnostic groups: 1) PackYears=pack-years of cigarette smoking, 2) Sand=sandblasting exposure, 3) q3g=walking more than one kilometer, and 4) q9i=tiredness during the past four weeks. Pack-years of cigarette smoking and months of sandblasting exposure were continuous measures. The categorical responses for 'Limitations in walking more than one kilometer were: all of the time, most of the time, some of the time, a little of the time, and none of the time. The categorical responses for 'tiredness' were yes, limited a lot; yes, limited a little; and no, not limited at all.

Figure 4. Classification and regression tree for the derivation sample (N=1,293) for an analysis without differential opportunity costs

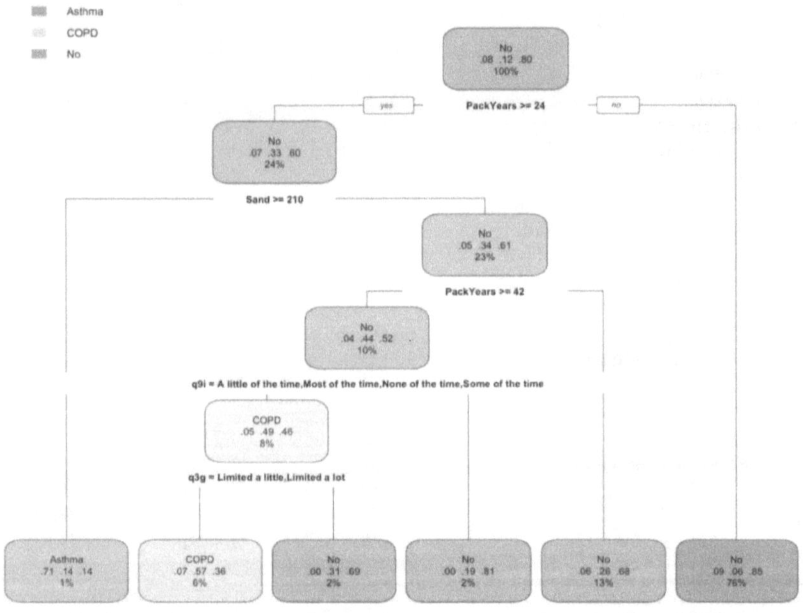

Each node displays the predictive class, predicted probabilities, and percentage of observations. Values in second row of each node are presented in alphabetical order of Asthma, COPD, and No OLD. Variables: q9i=During the past four weeks, how much of the time have you felt tired; q3g=Walking more than one kilometer; Sand=≥3 months of sandblasting exposure.

The first branching in the decision tree was for pack-years of smoking. Persons with less than 24 pack-years have an 85% predicted probability of not having OLD. Persons with more than 24 pack-years and more than 210 months of sandblasting exposure had a 71% predicted probability of asthma. A higher interaction was identified by the decision tree: persons with more than 42 pack-years, who responded yes to any of those four responses for tiredness, and were limited in walking more than one kilometer, had a 57% predicted probability of COPD. For the derivation model, a 3x3 confusion matrix is outputted and the sensitivity and specificity for each disease and no OLD was calculated, as shown in **Table 10**. When applying the tree to the derivation sample, correct classification occurred for 1001 of the 1028 cases of no OLD, 5 of the 109 cases of asthma, and 41 of the 156 cases of COPD. CART determines the predicted outcome of each decision node by the group with the highest predicted probability. The classification rate is determined by whether a participant falls in their true disease group based on their responses to those predictors. This CART analysis does not take into account the differential opportunity costs for prediction errors.

Table 10. Associated sensitivity and specificity for each disease in the derivation sample for a CART analysis without differential opportunity costs (N=1,293)[†]

Predicted Disease	True Disease			
	Asthma	COPD	No	Total
Asthma	5	1	1	7
COPD	5	41	26	72
No	99	114	1001	1214
Total	109	156	1028	N=1293
Sensitivity	5%	26%	97%	---
Specificity	99%	97%	20%	---

[†]The order of outcomes are presented in alphabetical order in R Studio Software (Asthma, COPD, No)

The AUC of the CART applied to the validation sample was 0.65 (95% CI: 0.52, 0.74) for COPD and 0.62 (95% CI: 0.60, 0.82) for asthma (**Figure 5**). When the tree was applied to the validation sample, the model correctly classified 10 of the 39 COPD cases; 247 of the 256 cases of no OLD; but none of the 27 asthma cases.

Figure 5. Receiver operator characteristic curves and corresponding AUC for the CART model in the validation sample: 0.65 for COPD and 0.62 for asthma (N=322). The analysis takes no account of differential opportunity costs.

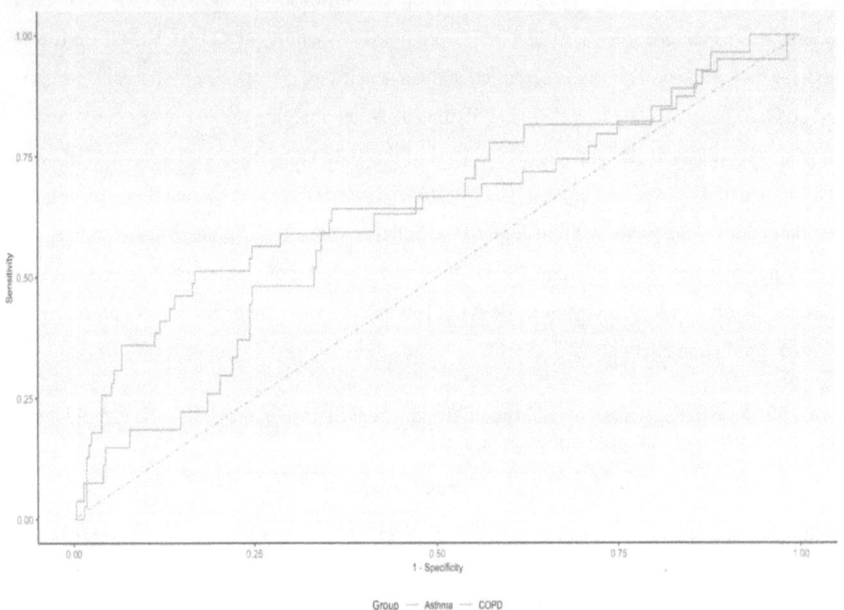

For classification and regression trees, the model determines the outcome (class) with the largest proportion. In this model, no OLD was considered the predictive class for most of the predictors. One challenge for CART and many other machine-learning algorithms is the class imbalance issue for multi-class outcomes (i.e., 8% versus 12% versus 80% for disease outcomes in this application). In addition, CART results have been known to be sensitive to peculiarities of the dataset and this quality may limit the robustness of the method when compared to logistic or linear regression models. With class imbalance, cases can be misclassified as being from the majority class, i.e., the no/negative outcome, which can increase the likelihood of false negatives.[151–154]

Alternative solutions have been proposed to address class imbalance, including changing the prior probabilities of each class, or over-sampling the minority class by duplicating the minority cases, in the derivation sample. However, prior probabilities and over-sampling were not used in this application to guard against overfitting the model.[151] A more appropriate remedy to class imbalance was to adopt a misclassification cost matrix since the matrix can be applied to input penalties on incorrect predictions directly when 'rpart' builds the tree.

Given the purpose of the book was to identify as many cases of OLD as possible because false negatives can result in relatively large societal costs, another decision tree was created to address the imbalance problem by taking account of the differential costs of prediction errors. The previous decision tree resulted in only four predictors (pack-years of cigarette smoking, sandblasting exposure, tiredness, and limitations walking more than one kilometre) with none containing any predictors related to symptoms of a respiratory disease. A second decision tree was created with the same misclassification costs applied to choose the risk cut-offs for the multinomial logistic regression model, i.e., a false negative for asthma incurred a cost of 10 units, a false negative for COPD incurred a cost of 8 units, and a false positive for OLD incurred a cost of 1 unit. Given 'rpart' outputs a 3x3 table instead of a 2x3, the cost of a false positive concluding a true Asthma case was COPD or a true COPD case was asthma was assigned a nominal small cost of 0.5 in the 'rpart' cost matrix.

3.3.1 Application of a Cost-Matrix

The decision tree with the misclassification costs applied is displayed in **Figure 6**. Compared to the other decision tree, three new predictors were found: 1) Age, in years, 2) Paint= months of paint, chemical and fume exposure, and 3) Wheezing in the morning. The pack-years of cigarette smoking and tiredness during the past four weeks were still retained as significant predictors. A matrix of the predicted versus true state of OLD for the derivation sample (**Table 11**) shows that the sensitivity values have increased for each disease.

Figure 6. Classification and regression tree of derivation sample with weights applied (N=1,293)[†]

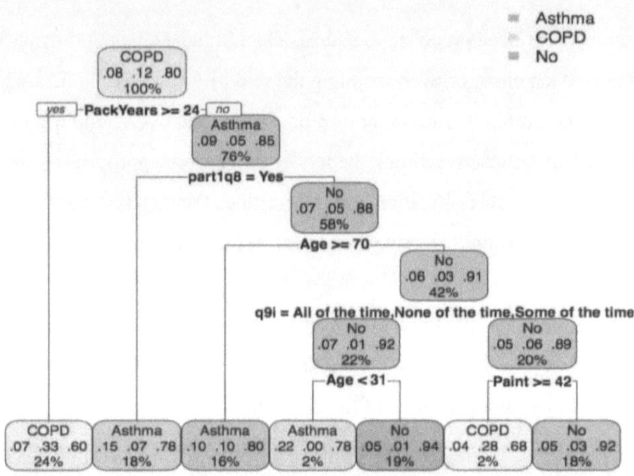

Each node displays the predictive class, predicted probabilities, and percentage of observations. Values in second row of each node are presented in alphabetical order of Asthma, COPD, and No OLD. Variables: part1q8=If you have a wheeze, it is worse in the morning; q9i= During the past four weeks, how much of the time have you felt tired; Paint=≥3 months of paint, chemical, or fume exposure.

Table 11. Application of cost weights in the CART analysis and the associated sensitivity and specificity for each disease in the derivation sample (N=1,293)[†]

Predicted Disease	True Disease			
	Asthma	COPD	No	Total
Asthma	63	37	372	472
COPD	21	109	205	335
No	25	10	451	486
Total	109	156	1028	N=1293
Sensitivity	58%	69%	44%	---
Specificity	75%	80%	87%	---

[†]The order of outcomes is presented in alphabetical order in R Studio Software (Asthma, COPD, No)

Applying the newly derived tree to the internal validation sample, the area under the ROC curve of the validation sample was 0.74 (95% CI: 0.66, 0.81) for COPD and 0.61 (95% CI: 0.49, 0.76) for asthma (**Figure 7**). The tree correctly classified 21 of the 39 COPD cases; 126 of the 256 cases of no OLD; and 13 of the 27 asthma cases in the validation sample. With the cost weights applied, correct classification occurred for 11 more cases of COPD and 13 cases of asthma were identified, whereas no cases of asthma were identified by the previous CART model.

Figure 7. Receiver operator characteristic curves and corresponding AUC for the CART model in the validation sample: 0.74 for COPD and 0.61 for asthma with cost weights applied (N=322)

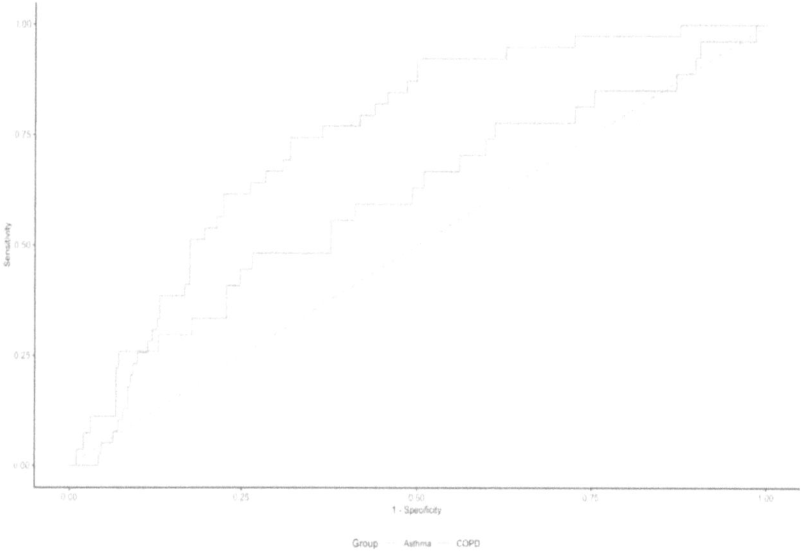

3.3.2 Comparison of Classification and Regression Tree and Multinomial Logistic Regression Models

A direct comparison of the multinomial logistic regression and CART models is hindered by the fact that their internal validation methods involve different sample sizes for the training and validation samples. The multinomial logistic regression model was internally validated with 10-fold cross validation while CART was internally validated with a one-time split into a derivation sample (N=1293) and a validation sample (N=322). The comparisons presented in Tables 12 and 13 should be interpreted with this limitation in mind.

Table 12. Comparison of AUC values for derivation and internal validation samples between the CART and multinomial logistic regression models

AUC	COPD		Asthma	
	CART	**Multinomial Logistic Regression**	**CART**	**Multinomial Logistic Regression**
Derivation	0.80	0.82	0.65	0.69
Internal Validation	0.74	0.79	0.61	0.64

Table 13. Application of the opportunity costs in the multinomial logistic regression and CART models

Method	True Asthma Cases Missed (Unit cost of 10)	True COPD Cases Missed (Unit cost of 8)	True No OLD Cases Misclassified (Unit cost of 1)	Total Cost	Sample Size	Average Cost per Person
MLR	12	7	1036	12(10)+7(8)+1036(1) =1212	1580	0.77
CART[1]	25	10	577	25(10)+10(8)+577(1) =907	1293	0.70

MLR=Multinomial Logistic Regression. [1]Cost calculation for CART ignores the small opportunity unit cost associated with predicting Asthma cases as COPD cases and vice versa; a unit cost is required by 'rpart'

The AUC values for the CART model in the derivation and the internal validation samples are similar, but the logistic regression performs moderately better, as shown in **Table 12**. **Table 13** was derived by applying the false negatives identified in Tables 7 and 11. The average cost per person is slightly less with the CART model. Although the cost-minimization exercise slightly favored the CART over the MLR model, the AUC results favored the multinomial logistic regression model over the CART. The MLR model was more sensitive than the CART model and missed fewer cases of undiagnosed asthma and COPD. In addition, the predictors (age; pack-years of cigarette smoking; paint, chemical, fume exposure; level of tiredness; and wheezing in the morning) in the CART model contained less disease-specific risk factors and is less clinically applicable compared to the multinomial logistic regression model. In terms of feasible applicability in the community, the interpretability of the model may not be as clear.[155,156]

Ultimately for these reasons, the MLR model was chosen as the preferred model. For the remaining analyses of the book, the UCAP Questionnaire will be based on the logistic regression model summarized in Tables 4 and 5.

3.4 Readability of the UCAP Questionnaire

The Flesch-Kincaid Grade Level was 7 and the Flesch-Kincaid Reading Ease score was 70.9, indicating "fairly easy" readability. The calculation was based solely on the 13 questions and corresponding answer choices.

3.5 Acceptability and Face Validity of the UCAP Questionnaire

Feedback about the UCAP Questionnaire was sought from samples of clinicians, study participants, and interviewers after model was derived. A total of 12 Respirologists and General Internists who care for patients with COPD and asthma, 27 UCAP study participants, and one interviewer provided feedback. As the questions adopted for the UCAP Questionnaire were taken from existing questionnaires, with only minor edits for formatting, this feedback is especially important in knowing what improvements might be achieved by rewording questions or revising the questionnaire structure. The feedback survey for clinicians and participants contained the following four questions, together with a closing open-ended section for comments and suggestions: 1) Was the wording of the questions clear, easy to understand, and interpret? If no, please elaborate. 2) Does the list of responses for each question feel adequate? If no, please elaborate. 3) How was the overall flow and structure of the questions? 4) Was the time to complete the questions reasonable? The responses for the survey from clinicians and participants are displayed in **Figure 8**.

Figure 8. Left graph illustrates UCAP participants' responses. Right graph illustrates clinicians' responses.

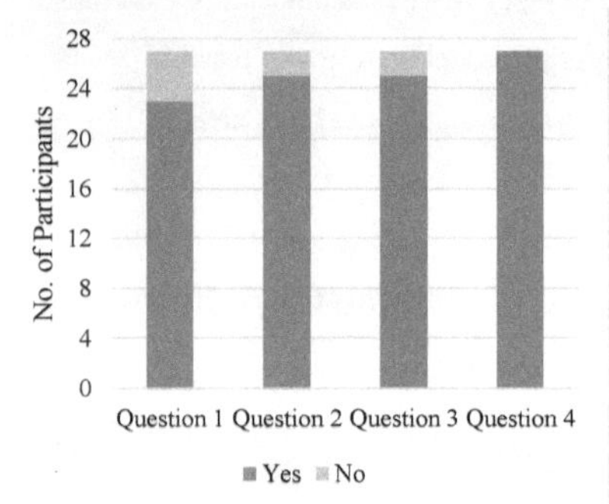

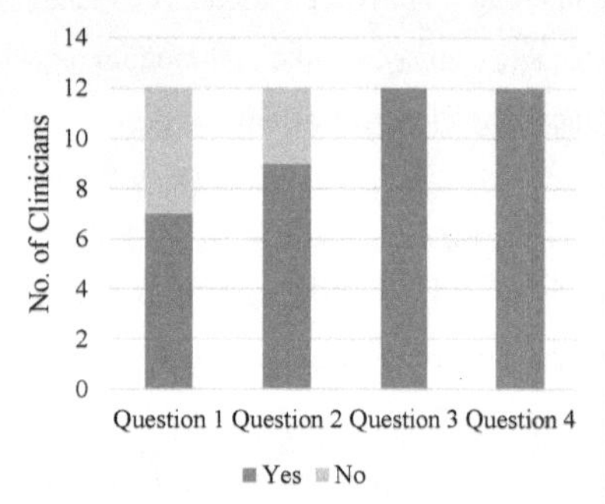

For question 1, regarding the clarity and interpretability of the questionnaire, five clinicians and four respondents specified concerns about some of the questions. Of the concerns specified, two were related to the length and syntax of question 13, "During the past 4 weeks, how much of the time have you had to cut down on the amount of time you spent on work or other regular activities as a result of any emotional problems, such as feeling depressed or anxious?" Some concerns were related to question 9, "Please rate your sleep on a scale of 0 to 5 with 0 meaning I sleep soundly to 5 meaning I do not sleep soundly because of my lung condition," The concern was that the soundness of sleep might be unrelated to lung condition. Two concerns were related to clarifying "chest problems" in question 7. Similar concerns were expressed for the sleep question by participants, i.e., ambiguity about whether the response should be related to lung condition or not.

Question 2, regarding the response scales, raised concerns among three clinicians and two participants. Specific concerns among clinicians were to add more scales to question 11 and consider adding another scale for frequency of chest tightness. The original chest tightness question refers to only the severity of chest tightness. One suggestion was creating a new variable specific to the frequency of chest tightness. Among respondents, similar concerns were expressed about adding more scales to the physical activity question, and coughing question. Compared to the other response scales, the physical activity question only had three responses: Limited a lot, Limited a little, and Not limited at all. Some participants wished to adopt the 1-5 scale of the other existing questions to the physical activity question as they felt that three choices were too narrow.

For question 3 about the overall flow and structure, two respondents had concerns: (1) to either omit or restructure the age question into categories, and (2) to omit the primary and second-hand cigarette smoke exposure question because of repetitiveness. The latter concern about the repetitiveness for the smoking question can be skipped if completed in-person, or the question can be skipped if the respondent is a current cigarette smoker. For the preliminary findings of the book, to adequately compare the derived model and the model evaluated in the external population, no more responses scales or new variables were added to the model, and age was kept as a continuous predictor.

Another set of questions was prepared for interviewers: 1) Was the script clear and adequate for the interview? 2) Did you need to explain any questions or elaborate unduly on response options? 3) Please estimate the time required to complete the questionnaire, and 4) Do you have any other comments or suggestions? For the interviewer-administered questions, the script was found to be clear and adequate. The interviewer reported six of the 27 participants required elaboration about the sleep question, i.e., only if related to lung condition. The average time to complete the questions by telephone was approximately six minutes.

Modifications were made to clarify any clinical ambiguity around the questions, specifically for chest problems, in which 'chest problems' refers to wheeze, shortness of breath. For, "Please rate your sleep on a scale of 0 to 5 with 0 meaning I sleep soundly to 5 meaning I do not sleep soundly only because of my lung condition," the word 'only' was added to the question.

3.6 Test-retest Reliability

A total of 41 consenting participants from the UCAP study were telephoned for test-retest, of which 27 completed the administration of the questionnaire at two time points one-week apart.

The mean of the differences (between time one and time two) and the limits of agreement are presented in **Table 14**. The Bland-Altman plots are shown for pack-years of smoking and paint, chemical, and fume exposure in **Figures 9** and **10**. From the plots, approximately 95% of the differences fall inside the limits of agreement. The test-retest responses for the smoking and occupational variables were frequently identical because most participants were non-smokers (zero pack-years) and were never exposed to occupational paint, chemicals, or fumes, i.e., zero exposure. Consequently, most mean differences between responses at the two time points were close to zero.

Table 14. Mean response differences for UCAP Questionnaire participants at two time points one-week apart (N=27)

Question	Mean of Difference (95% CI)	Lower LoA (95% CI)	Upper LoA (95% CI)
How old are you?	-0.07 (-0.18, 0.03)	-0.60 (-0.78, 0.41)	0.50 (0.26, 0.63)
Are you currently smoking cigarettes or have you smoked cigarettes in the past? If yes, calculate total pack-years.	-1.16 (-4.76, 2.44)	-19.01 (-25.2, -12.77)	16.69 (10.46, 22.93)
Have you ever worked for 3 months or more with paint, chemicals, or fumes? If yes, how many months did you work?	15.55 (-16.42, 47.53	-142.9 (-198.2, -87.54)	173.9 (118.6, 229.3)

†LoA = Limits of agreement

Figure 9. Bland-Altman plot for pack-years of cigarette smoking. A plot of the mean response difference against the average response at time 1 and time 2. Dashed lines represent the upper LoA (16.69) and lower LoA (-19.01) and the central line represents the mean of -1.16.

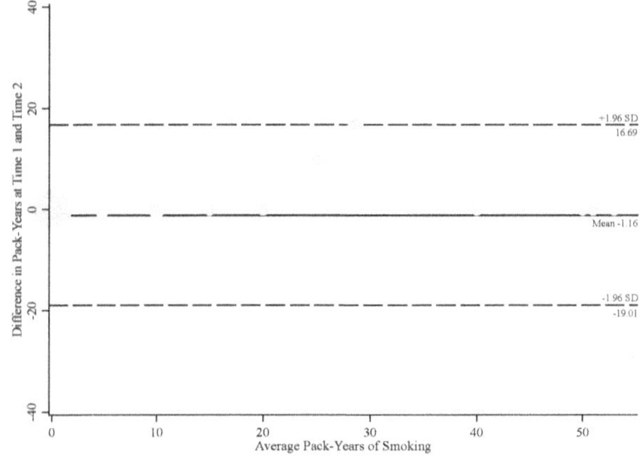

Figure 10. Bland-Altman plot for exposure of paint, chemical, or fumes in months. A plot of the mean response difference against the average response at time 1 and time 2. Dashed lines represent the upper LoA (173.9) and lower LoA (-142.9) and the central line represents the mean of 15.55.

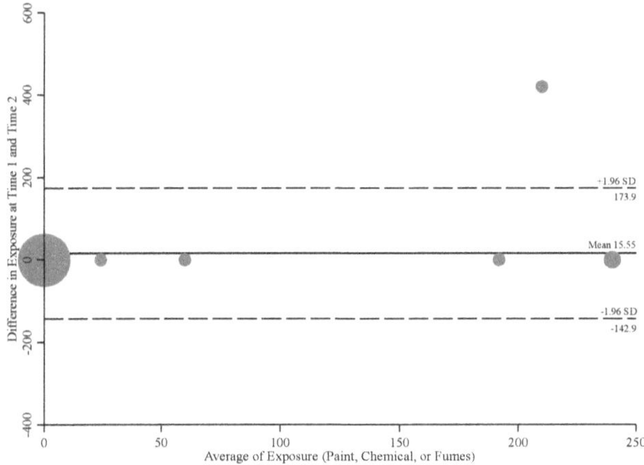

Figure 11. Frequency of test-retest shifts on selected ordinal UCAP Questionnaire items, sorted by ascending number of categories of no response shift (N=27)

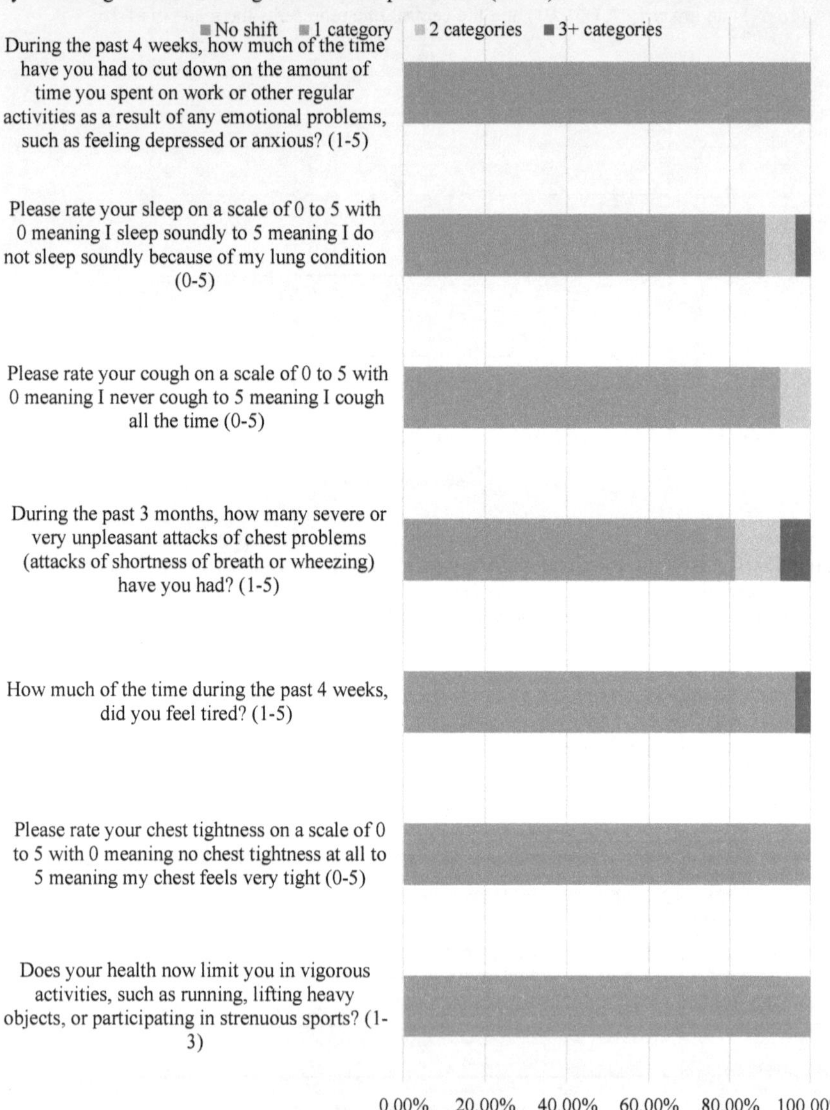

No shift
1 category
2 categories
3+ categories
During the past 4 weeks, how much of the time have you had to cut down on the amount of time you spent on work or other regular activities as a result of any emotional problems, such as feeling depressed or anxious? (1-5)
Please rate your sleep on a scale of 0 to 5 with 0 meaning I sleep soundly to 5 meaning I do not sleep soundly because of my lung condition (0-5)
Please rate your cough on a scale of 0 to 5 with 0 meaning I never cough to 5 meaning I cough all the time (0-5)
During the past 3 months, how many severe or very unpleasant attacks of chest problems (attacks of shortness of breath or wheezing) have you had? (1-5)
How much of the time during the past 4 weeks, did you feel tired? (1-5)
Please rate your chest tightness on a scale of 0 to 5 with 0 meaning no chest tightness at all to 5 meaning my chest feels very tight (0-5)
Does your health now limit you in vigorous activities, such as running, lifting heavy objects, or participating in strenuous sports? (1-3)
0.00%
20.00%
40.00%
60.00%
80.00%
100.00%

Table 15. Test retest reliability of the UCAP Questionnaire (N=27)

Question	ICC	95% CI
How old are you?	0.999	0.999-0.999
Are you currently smoking cigarettes or have you smoked cigarettes in the past? If yes, calculate total pack-years.	0.895	0.783-0.951
Have you ever worked for 3 months or more with paint, chemicals, or fumes? If yes, how many months did you work?	0.592	0.280-0.790
Have you ever worked for 3 months or more with sandblasting? If yes, how many months did you work?	1.00	1.00-1.00
	Weighted Kappa	**95% CI**
Are you regularly exposed to cigarette smoke (either from yourself, or from people around you) on a daily basis?	1.00[†]	1.00-1.00
Are you currently taking the medication Salbutamol (also known as Ventolin) for your breathing?	1.00[†]	1.00-1.00
If you have a wheeze, is it worse in the morning?	1.00[†]	1.00-1.00
During the past 3 months, how many severe or very unpleasant attacks of chest problems (attacks of shortness of breath or wheezing) have you had?	0.763	0.528-0.999
Please rate your cough on a scale of 0 to 5 with 0 meaning I never cough to 5 meaning I cough all the time.	0.877	0.766-0.987
Please rate your sleep on a scale of 0 to 5 with 0 meaning I sleep soundly to 5 meaning I do not sleep soundly only because of my lung condition.	0.871	0.745-0.996
Please rate your chest tightness on a scale of 0 to 5 with 0 meaning no chest tightness at all to 5 meaning my chest feels very tight.	0.929	0.845-1.00
Does your health now limit you in vigorous activities, such as running, lifting heavy objects, or participating in strenuous sports?	0.923	0.825-1.00
How much of the time during the past 4 weeks, did you feel tired?	0.739	0.399-1.00
During the past 4 weeks, how much of the time have you had to cut down on the amount of time you spent on work or other regular activities as a result of any emotional problems, such as feeling depressed or anxious?	0.853	0.749-0.956

[†]Unweighted Kappa

Table 16. Test retest reliability of the UCAP Questionnaire stratified by age (N=27)

Question	Age ≤64 years N=14		Age ≥65 years N=13	
	ICC	95% CI	ICC	95% CI
How old are you?	0.999	0.998-0.999	1.00	1.00-1.00
Are you currently smoking cigarettes or have you smoked cigarettes in the past? If yes, calculate total pack-years.	0.972	0.915-0.991	0.837	0.564-0.947
Have you ever worked for 3 months or more with paint, chemicals, or fumes? If yes, how many months did you work?	0.258	-0.285-0.679	1.00	1.00-1.00
Have you ever worked for 3 months or more with sandblasting? If yes, how many months did you work?	1.00	1.00-1.00	--	--
	Weighted Kappa	**95% CI**	**Weighed Kappa**	**95% CI**
Are you regularly exposed to cigarette smoke (either from yourself, or from people around you) on a daily basis?	1.00[†]	1.00-1.00	1.00[†]	1.00-1.00
Are you currently taking the medication Salbutamol (also known as Ventolin) for your breathing?	1.00[†]	1.00-1.00	1.00[†]	1.00-1.00
If you have a wheeze, is it worse in the morning?	1.00[†]	1.00-1.00	1.00[†]	1.00-1.00
During the past 3 months, how many severe or very unpleasant attacks of chest problems (attacks of shortness of breath or wheezing) have you had?	0.793	0.515-1.00	0.763	0.527-0.999
Please rate your cough on a scale of 0 to 5 with 0 meaning I never cough to 5 meaning I cough all the time.	0.871	0.717-1.00	0.867	0.690-1.00
Please rate your sleep on a scale of 0 to 5 with 0 meaning I sleep soundly to 5 meaning I do not sleep soundly only because of my lung condition.	0.885	0.685-1.00	0.849	0.697-1.00
Please rate your chest tightness on a scale of 0 to 5 with 0 meaning no chest tightness at all to 5 meaning my chest feels very tight.	0.947	0.888-1.00	0.901	0.703-1.00
Does your health now limit you in vigorous activities, such as running, lifting heavy objects, or participating in strenuous sports?	1.00	1.00-1.00	0.852	0.598-1.00

| How much of the time during the past 4 weeks, did you feel tired? | 0.964 | 0.885-1.00 | 0.277 | -0.599-1.00 |
| During the past 4 weeks, how much of the time have you had to cut down on the amount of time you spent on work or other regular activities as a result of any emotional problems, such as feeling depressed or anxious? | 0.848 | 0.716-0.981 | 0.824 | 0.609-1.00 |

†Unweighted Kappa

The frequency distributions of categorical response shifts for ordinal variables are displayed in **Figure 11**. Most participants had either no response shift, or a shift to the adjacent category. Three of the variables (sleep, chest problems, and tiredness) did have shifts of three or more categories between the time points for one or more participants.

The Kappa and ICC values are presented in **Table 15**. "Excellent" agreement and "almost perfect" agreement (0.739-1.00) were reported for age, pack-years of cigarette smoke, second-hand smoke exposure, use of salbutamol, wheeze, cough, sleep, chest tightness, physical activity limitation, and emotional health. "Substantial" agreement was found among chest problems and tiredness. Only "moderate" agreement (0.592) was found for paint, fume, and chemical exposure; however, this ICC is influenced by a very large difference in responses between time points for one participant. Figure 10 shows this 420-month difference.

Subgroup analyses of the ICCs by age (**Table 16**) found the group under 65 years tended to yield higher ICC values; however, most of the results are comparable between the two age groupings except for the level of tiredness and the paint exposure question. The question about tiredness had higher reliability for those under 65 years (0.964) compared to 0.277 for those over 65 years. For the occupational paint exposure question, the group over 65 years had excellent reliability (1.00) compared to the 0.258 for the group under 65 years.

Given the changes in some of the responses in the one-week interval, **Figure 12** was used to illustrate the differences in risk probabilities between time one and time two for each of the diseases. Of specific interest was whether the eligibility status (eligible if risk probability was greater than or equal to 6%) changed as a result of the different responses. In two of the participants, the changes in their responses had switched their status from "Ineligible" to "Eligible." The differences between test and retest were 3.54% and 5.00% for these two participants.

Figure 12. Scatterplot of the differences of the predicted probability of each disease between time 1 and time 2 (N=27)

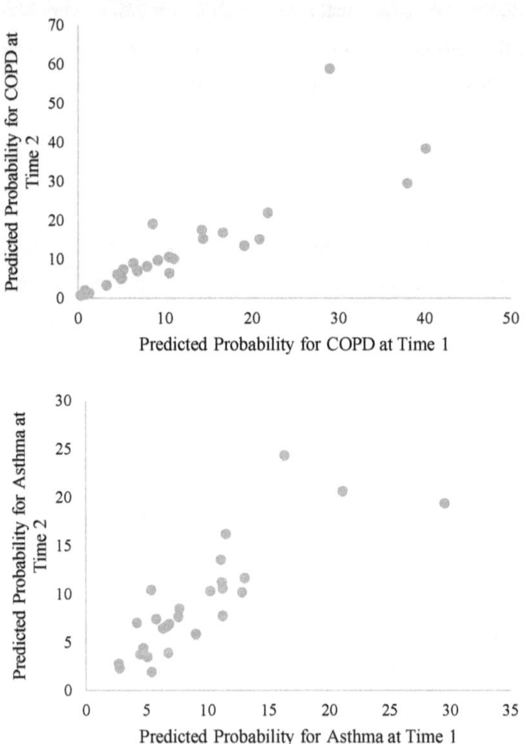

3.7 External Validation of the UCAP Questionnaire

A total of 74 participants were recruited for the validation study from October 2020 to January 2021, of which eight were ultimately diagnosed with asthma and six were ultimately diagnosed with COPD. **Table 17** shows the characteristics of the validation cohort. Compared to the derivation cohort, median age for asthma was younger (53 years versus 60 years) and non-smokers were more prevalent than current or former smokers in the asthma group.

Table 17. Demographic and clinical characteristics of validation cohort (N=74)

Characteristics	No obstructive lung disease (OLD) N=60	Asthma N=8	COPD N=6
Age, year[†]	65 (54-75)	53 (24-70)	67 (64-76)
Sex (n, %)			
Female	38 (64)	3 (38)	2 (33)
Male	21 (36)	5 (63)	4 (67)
Race/Ethnicity (n, %)			
Caucasian	59 (98)	8 (100)	6 (100)
Black or African American	1 (2)	0	0
Level of education (n, %)			
High school or less	15 (25)	3 (38)	1 (17)
Some college/university	14 (23)	1 (13)	3 (50)
College/university	31 (52)	4 (50)	2 (33)
Smoking history (n, %)			
Current	8 (13)	3 (38)	1 (17)
Former	22 (37)	1 (13)	3 (50)
Never	30 (50)	4 (50)	2 (33)
Occupational exposure (n, %)			
Yes	18 (30)	1 (13)	1 (17)
No	70 (42)	7 (88)	5 (83)
Pre-bronchodilator spirometry[†]			
FEV_1	2.51 (1.92-3.07)	2.75 (1.94-4.08)	1.91 (1.45-2.42)
FEV_1 % predicted	97 (88-111)	84 (69-95)	71 (47-78)
FEV_1/FVC	77 (73-80)	67 (65-75)	58 (43-65)
Post-bronchodilator spirometry[†]			
FEV_1	2.62 (1.99-3.11)	3.09 (2.26-4.59)	1.96 (1.54-2.50)
FEV_1 % predicted	100 (90-113)	98 (78-105)	72 (51-80)
FEV_1/FVC	79 (74-82)	73 (69-81)	59 (49-63)

[†]Data are presented as median (P25-P75)

To assess the validity of the UCAP Questionnaire, sensitivity and specificity values, and the AUC were used to evaluate the case-finding tool in comparison to the ASQ and COPD-DQ. A 2x3 table was created to assess the sensitivity, specificity, PPV, and NPV of the UCAP Questionnaire, ASQ, and COPD-DQ using the multinomial outcome with their respective risk cut-offs (**Tables 18** and **19**). At a cut-off of 6%, the sensitivity of the questionnaire for diagnosing either COPD or asthma was 100%; specificity was 13%; PPV was 23%; and NPV was 100%. For the ASQ and COPD-DQ combined, the sensitivity of the questionnaires for diagnosing COPD was 100%; sensitivity for diagnosing asthma was 50%; specificity was 28%; PPV was 19%; and NPV was 81%. In summary, the UCAP Questionnaire identified four additional asthma cases than the COPD-DQ and ASQ combined, at the cost of nine false positives. Using the external validation sample, the AUC for asthma was 0.65 (95% CI: 0.63-0.72) and the AUC for COPD was 0.89 (95% CI: 0.62-0.90), shown in **Figure 13** and **14**, respectively. The "number needed to treat" (NNT) was another measure calculated to determine the number of people needed to be treated to prevent one adverse outcome. Most often, the NNT is used to express the results of clinical trials. The NNT is the reciprocal of the absolute risk reduction, the difference in event rate between the experimental (Group 'Yes') and control (Group 'No') group. Based on Table 18, in order to prevent one adverse outcome, five people would need to be treated.

Table 18. Classification table of predicted OLD against the true state of disease for the external validation sample basing on screening that used the UCAP Questionnaire

	UCAP Questionnaire		
	True Disease[††]		
Prediction of OLD at a risk cut-off of ≥6%[†]	**COPD**	**Asthma**	**No OLD**	**Total**
Yes	6	8	52	66
No	0	0	8	8
Total	6	8	60	N=74

[†]OLD is predicted if the risk probability for either disease is greater or equal to 6% [††]Gold standard reference of spirometry [††]Gold standard reference of spirometry

Table 19. Classification table of predicted OLD against the true state of disease for the external validation sample based on screening that used the ASQ and COPD-DQ

	ASQ & COPD-DQ			
	True Disease[††]			
Prediction of OLD at a risk cut-off of ≥6 or >19.5[†]	**COPD**	**Asthma**	**No OLD**	**Total**
Yes	6	4	43	53
No	0	4	17	21
Total	6	8	60	N=74

ASQ: Asthma Screening Questionnaire; COPD-DQ: COPD Diagnostic Questionnaire [†]ASQ score of 6 or more or COPD-DQ score of 19.5 or more [††]Gold standard reference of spirometry

Figure 13. Receiver operating characteristic curve for UCAP Questionnaire for diagnosing asthma. AUC=0.65.

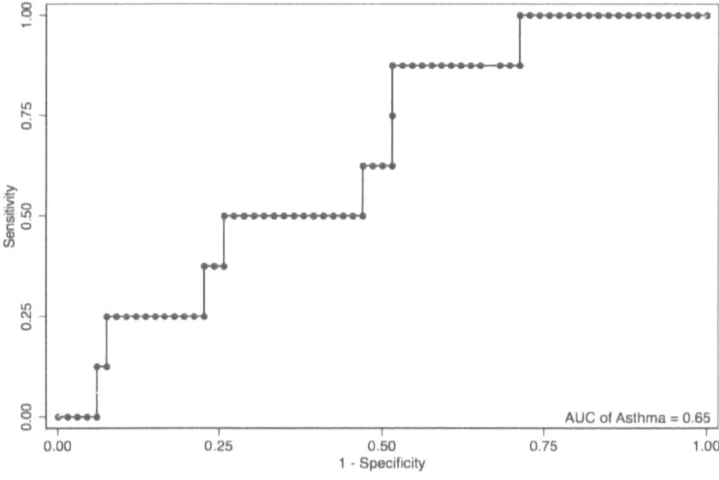

Figure 14. Receiver operating characteristic curve for UCAP Questionnaire for diagnosing COPD. AUC=0.89.

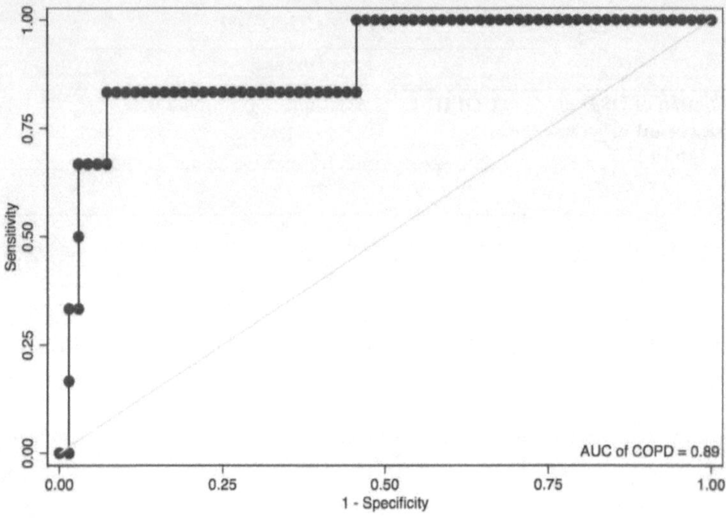

<h1 align="center">4. Discussion</h1>

This book sought to develop and validate a case-finding questionnaire to identify undiagnosed lung disease in symptomatic community-dwelling adults. To date, this marks the first study to combine both asthma and COPD diseases into a single case-finding instrument. A single instrument is appropriate because the two diseases, although they are distinct in terms of their pathophysiology, have many symptoms in common. This book contributes to the case-finding literature by creating a short, practical and effective survey instrument for identifying persons with obstructive airflow limitation.

Based on the multinomial logistic regression model, 13 questions were found to be jointly predictive of disease: age in years, number of pack-years of cigarette smoke, primary or second-hand smoking exposure, cough, sleep, chest tightness, number of chest problems, symptoms of wheeze in the morning, tiredness during the past four weeks, ≥3 months of paint exposure, ≥3 months sandblasting exposure, physical activity limitations, and use of salbutamol. The model demonstrated modest discriminative ability for COPD (AUC of 0.82, 95% CI: 0.78-0.86), but a lower discriminative ability for asthma (AUC of 0.69, 95% CI: 0.64-0.74).

4.1 Strengths in Comparison to Existing Case-Finding and Screening Instruments

The predictors contained in the final model are consistent with previously published instruments found in Sections 1.61 (compared in **Table 20**) and 1.62. While not as commonly found in the other case-finding instruments, this study incorporated second-hand smoke exposure, sleep, emotional health, and occupational exposure (specific to chemicals, fumes, painting and sandblasting) as predictors for undiagnosed lung disease. These questions serve as a strength because they represent risk factors related to wellness and environmental factors. For instance, sleep disturbance or poor quality of sleep has been cited as a frequently reported symptom among OLD patients;[157–159] higher prevalence of depression, fatigue, and anxiety among patients diagnosed with OLD;[160,161] and, the increased risk of asthma from occupational exposures have been shown in several studies.[162,163] It is worthwhile to mention this study found no significant association with participants' sex or the presence of phlegm. Another predictor found in the COPD-DQ and the Sà-Sousa et al. study was a history of allergies, but this predictor was not available in this dataset. The predictive performance for COPD was comparable with existing COPD instruments, which range from 0.64 to 0.82. In comparison to the handful of adult asthma questionnaires, which had AUCs between 0.75 to a high 0.913, the predictive performance of the UCAP Questionnaire was lower. However, these asthma questionnaires were not externally validated and were tested with relatively small sample sizes. The A2 and GALEN questionnaires included questions that were attempting to discriminate between participants with and without asthma, e.g., ever had a physician-diagnosis of asthma, currently have asthma, and having an asthma attack in the last 12 months. In addition, some of these existing case-finding studies had derived and validated their instrument with participants already diagnosed with OLD. In comparison to the UCAP study, participants with a prior physician diagnosis of OLD were omitted to assess the instrument with a more representative population.

The existing case-finding instruments were described earlier as having methodological flaws related to the diagnostic criteria, sample size for derivation, and lack of external validation. This study aimed to address some of these limitations by confirming obstructive airflow with spirometry rather than a self-reported diagnosis and using the lower limit of the 95% confidence interval for healthy participants (matched for sex, age and height) to reduce misclassification. The major strengths of this study were the large sample size for model derivation, the use of multiple sites, representative samples recruited at the sites by random-digit dialing, validation of the model using an external independent sample, and assessment of reliability. The other case-finding tools were often developed by using data from pulmonary clinics, primary care clinics, or including previously diagnosed participants. Hence the high predictive performance measures (e.g., PPV, NPV) were likely a reflection of the increased disease prevalence in a selected population.[115–117] Data obtained for this study, however, were gathered by random sampling of the general adult population and the prevalence rate obtained in this study for each disease (i.e., 8 and 12%) is likely to be a more representative estimate of the current prevalence of undiagnosed asthma and COPD in Canada.

The validity of study findings is closely associated with the quality of the data and execution of the study. Compared to other study designs, this final case-finding tool was derived from a set of five published questionnaires (CAT, ASQ, WPAIGH, SF-36 QoL, SGRQ) and one study-specific collection form, the Personal Information Sheet. This derivation strategy was considered a strength as these questionnaires included non-clinical predictors, such as quality of life and days lost from work due to breathing problems, that are not documented in electronic health records or health registries.

In terms of building the model, automated predictor selection was considered a reasonable method of choice given the sheer volume of screening variables. Automated variable selection has frequent application in model-building and is effective at reducing a sizable quantity of variables to a smaller subset.[135,164] Despite the advantages of using a backward elimination algorithm, automated predictor selection has been previously cited in the literature as being prone to biased coefficients, p-values and standard errors, vulnerable to excessive multicollinearity as some software programs can have all variables enter, and, can lead to model-building practices dependent exclusively on statistical associations and without review of clinical plausibility.[165] To ensure the best predictors in this study, different criteria were applied including clinical judgement, review of the literature, and preliminary univariate statistical significance testing to create a candidate pool of predictors, rather than inputting *all* predictors and relying on the statistical significance filtering of the algorithm alone.

The statistical software used for variable selection protects against collinearity between predictors, but a manual review of the variables was assessed as well. To add to the strength of this study, a secondary model-building technique was performed with recursive partitioning using CART. Of the two models, the logistic regression model was considered the more appropriate model of choice based on feasibility of implementation and valuable disease-specific risk factors.

Table 20. Comparison of predictors and predictive performance between the UCAP Questionnaire and existing case-finding or screening COPD instrument

Predictors	UCAP Questionnaire	LFQ	Could It Be COPD?	TargetCOPD	COPD-DQ	COPD-PS	PUMA Study	CAPTURE Study	COPD Scale
Demographic and Clinical Information	Age; Use of salbutamol	Age	Age ≥ 40	Age; Use of antibiotics or salbutamol	Age; Body mass index; History of allergies	Age	Age; Sex		Age
Smoking and Occupational Exposure	Pack-years of cigarette smoking; Primary or second-hand smoking; ≥3-month exposure to sandblasting or paint/chemical/fumes	Smoked for >20 years	Smoking status and pack-years of cigarette smoking	Smoking status		Smoking	Smoking	Exposure to air pollutants, dust, smoke, second-hand smoke	Pack-years of cigarette smoking
Symptoms	Chest tightness; Cough; Wheeze; Attacks of chest problems (e.g., shortness of breath)	Wheeze; Phlegm; Breathlessness	Cough; Phlegm; Breathlessness	Dyspnea	Weather-dependent Cough; Wheeze; Phlegm	Phlegm; Shortness of breath	Cough; Phlegm; Dyspnea	Breathing during different seasons	
Physical and Mental Wellness	Limitation of activities; Tiredness; Sleep; Emotional health					Limitation of activities		Limitation of activities; Easily tired	
Miscellaneous							Previous spirometry	Days of missed work, school or activities due to respiratory event	

Predictive Performance	UCAP Questionnaire	LFQ	Could It Be COPD?	TargetCOPD	COPD-DQ	COPD-PS	PUMA Study	CAPTURE Study	COPD Scale
Risk cut-off	$\geq$6%	$\geq$3	3 & $\geq$35 years old	$\geq$7.5	19.5	$\geq$5	$\geq$5	$\geq$2	$\geq$10
AUC	0.82	0.65	--	0.74	0.82	0.81	0.76	0.795	0.64
Sensitivity (%)	91	77.8	80.8	68.8	80.4	84.4	76.3	95.7	82.0
Specificity (%)	18	52.4	62.8	68.8	57.5	60.7	69.3	44.4	47.0
PPV (%)	23	--	32.7	14.4	30.3	56.8	38.5	--	--
NPV (%)	92	--	93.6	96.6	92.7	86.4	92.1	--	--

Based on the readability and feedback results, the case-finding tool contained valid predictors and was regarded as easy-to-read. The Flesch-Kincaid Reading Ease and Flesch-Kincaid Grade Level are objective measures to calculate readability as the formula is based on a sum of words, sentences, and syllables. One of the shortcomings of the Flesch-Kincaid, however, is that they do not truly capture comprehensiveness of a text, and, they do not measure other factors affecting reading ease, e.g., cultural context, knowledge of medical terms, fatigue. As a result, obtaining feedback from a representative sample and from clinicians were valuable, since research and practical experience show that expert reviews can help to identify problems with questions, face validity, clarity of questions, order of questions, and other concerns. Similarly, reviews by participants provide feedback from persons representative of the underlying target population. The general consensus was that the questionnaire flowed well and questions were mostly clear and interpretable. Participants and clinicians did have some concerns about specific questions, including wording of the sleep question and the definition of chest attacks. These issues were remedied with minor changes (as per Stewart's criteria describing modifications in survey design). No substantial modifications to the instrument were made.[166]

Repeated administration of the questionnaire among a volunteer sample of respondents showed stable responses over a one-week test interval. Of the 13 predictors, 12 predictors had ICCs ranging from 0.739 to 1.00. The lowest ICC (0.592) was attributed to the paint, fumes, and chemical exposure question. This sharply lower ICC was linked to a 420-month difference between time points for a single respondent as the ICC can be influenced by large differences. A one-week interval was selected to minimize carryover effects of recall and any actual changes occurring in health. That said, given the questions about number of severe chest problems and tiredness had only "substantial" test-retest agreement, real changes in health and symptoms may have occurred during the one-week interval. The Kappa value for the tiredness question among the 65 years and older group was smaller, reflecting greater shifts in responses between the time points. It is possible that other factors also could have influenced the test-retest findings, such as situational distractions, illness, and fatigue.

4.2 Limitations

As with any research study, this one has a few noteworthy limitations. First, the sample size used for external validation was lower than desired because of its dependence on recruitment in the ongoing UCAP study, which was interrupted by the COVID-19 pandemic. The book time frame dictated an abbreviated external validation. Different guidelines have been proposed for sample size calculation, with some studies suggesting a minimum of 100 events and 100 non-events for external validation.[167,168] The sample collected for the validation exercise was smaller than the estimate based on the desired precision of the AUC and smaller than the suggested minimum. Since the results are likely to be underpowered to adequately detect differences in predictive performance, the results in this study should be interpreted only as exploratory until more data are collected. In the absence of a large independent sample, internal cross-validation is a good alternative measure of performance. The average AUCs from the 10-fold cross validation were relatively similar to the model AUCs, thus supporting the internal validity of the model.

A second limitation is the ethnic homogeneity of the study population. Most of the derivation cohort (1493/1615, 93%) and validation cohort (73/74, 98%) was of one ethnic descent, suggesting only one subset of the population was well-represented. Given that the data gathered for this study was based on random digit dialing, only persons with access to a phone or a landline inside a 90-minute radius of the 16 study sites who wished to volunteer were included. Hence, rural or remote communities, shelters and institutions, locations extending beyond the 16 sites, and those who declined to participate were not captured in the UCAP data. In terms of the heterogeneity of the data, literature on the ethnic and racial profile of adult Canadians who have significant breathing limitations remains sparse. In contrast, recent research in the United States has assessed the racial/ethnic disparities in the prevalence of each disease.[169,170] Thus, the findings of this book highlight the need for further validation to assess the usefulness of the case-finding tool in different subpopulations.

Finally, the study has the potential for self-reporting bias. With interviewer-administered surveys, social desirability bias could have been possible, which occurs when participants respond in a manner deemed favorable to the researcher.[171] It is noted that social desirability bias tends to present with sensitive questions, e.g., income, level of education, mental health, health risk behaviors, and can vary based on different modes of administration, e.g., face-to-face, via telephone, or self-administered.[172] For derivation of the model, this bias could obscure or create a new predictor-outcome relationship due to under-reported or over-reported responses.[171] It is difficult to truly ascertain the magnitude of self-reporting bias in this application. Self-reported bias could have affected the risk probabilities during reliability testing and external validation. For test-retest, responses at two time points may be stable but there is no assurance that the responses are factual or accurate.

4.3 Implications and Future Directions

The current findings have implications for both clinical management and research. The UCAP Questionnaire was shown to be reliable and feasible. Undiagnosed lung disease remains a complex and multifactorial issue with barriers related to spirometry accessibility and self-awareness of symptoms. With its moderate accuracy for disease detection and applicability with the web-based calculator, the UCAP Questionnaire offers potential as part of a case-finding approach. The predictors in this model contain well-known predictors for lung disease, such as cough, smoking and wheeze, and with the advantage of questions derived from the SF-36 and SGRQ QoL tools, other strong predictors related to occupational exposure, fatigue, and emotional health were included. Given this questionnaire has only been externally validated in a small sample, prospective evaluation with the UCAP study is still ongoing to recruit a larger sample to re-evaluate the predictive performance. Moreover, the cost-benefits of the case-finding tool will be explored in another phase of the UCAP study.

This study has uniquely combined two obstructive lung diseases into a single case-finding tool and has provided insight into potential avenues to be explored. External validation in various settings (e.g., primary care) and subpopulations are still needed to evaluate the performance. The current case-finding strategy in this study has been recruiting participants within a specific radius of the study sites using the UCAP Questionnaire via telephone. However, alternative case-finding strategies with practical access to spirometry to identify larger numbers of undiagnosed cases should be assessed in future works. For instance, other case-finding approaches could use the UCAP questionnaire tool in primary care clinics, public spaces, rural communities, or community shelters to identify subjects within these settings with undiagnosed asthma or COPD. With the web-based calculator, the UCAP questionnaire can be administered in primary care offices, emailed to subjects, or made available online. However, if the questionnaire were to be disseminated in a paper-based form, a simplified version of the risk score may need to be generated. Even more, translating and validating this tool in different languages may aid future distribution. Future research should continue to evaluate the inclusion of other predictors for undiagnosed OLD, and even qualitative-based studies, such as interviews, to enable patients to share their perspectives and personal barriers to diagnosis. The association of prenatal and hereditary factors, such as childhood respiratory infections, premature birth, and maternal smoking exposure, have been highlighted in literature as robust risk factors. While these predictors were not available in this dataset, future studies should consider their inclusion to accurately detect persons with undiagnosed OLD and those potentially at-risk.

5. Conclusion

This book developed and validated a 13-item case-finding questionnaire useful for detecting undiagnosed OLD. The items included age, number of pack-years of cigarette smoke, primary or second-hand smoking exposure, cough, sleep, chest tightness, number of chest problems, symptoms of wheeze in the morning, tiredness during the past four weeks, ≥ 3 months of paint exposure, ≥ 3 months sandblasting exposure, physical activity limitations, and use of salbutamol. The findings from internal validation showed modest predictive ability for detecting asthma and COPD cases. This study does demonstrate the complex nature of identifying risk factors for undiagnosed adult lung disease, specifically for asthma. Future studies are required to continue validating the tool for use in different populations and in different clinical settings to capture the predictive ability of the questionnaire to case-find undiagnosed subjects with asthma or COPD.

Appendix A – List of Questionnaires

Questions from the following five questionnaires were used as potential predictors in building the case-finding questionnaire:

Personal Information Sheet
1. Age, years
2. Sex
3. Race/Ethnicity
4. Education
5. Income
6. Have you ever worked for 3 months or more at any of the following occupations? Hard-rock mining, coal mining, sandblasting, working with asbestos, chemical or plastics manufacturing, flour, feed or grain milling, cotton or jute processing, foundry or steel milling, welding, firefighting, farming, forestry, saw-milling, work with paint, chemicals, or fumes
7. Are you regularly exposed to any of the following on a daily basis?
    a. Smoking (primary or second-hand)
    b. Pets (dogs, cats, or fur animals)
8. Are you currently smoking cigarettes?
9. Have you every smoked pot/marijuana?
10. Have you ever tried an electronic cigarette, also known as an e-cigarette?
11. The last time you used an e-cigarette, did it contain nicotine?
12. In the past two years, did you ever use the e-cigarette as an aid while attempting to quit smoking?
13. Do you have a history of any of the following medical conditions?
14. Do you have a family doctor?
15. Can you see your family doctor within a week of requesting an appointment?
16. What is the distance in kms from your home to your family doctor?
17. Did you ever discuss your respiratory symptoms with a doctor?
18. Did any doctor give you an alternative diagnosis for your respiratory symptoms?
19. Did any doctor refer you to a specialist for your respiratory symptoms?
20. Did you ever have any of the following procedures for your respiratory symptoms?
21. In the past 12 months, did you visit your general practitioner or a nurse practitioner or another physician at a walk-in clinic for any breathing problems?
22. In the past 12 months, did you visit an emergency practitioner or a nurse practitioner or another physician at a walk-in clinic for any breathing problem?
23. In the past 12 months, did you visit an emergency department for any breathing problems?
24. In the past 12 months, were you hospitalized for any breathing problems or respiratory illness?
25. Are you currently taking any medications for your breathing?
26. Did you work in the past 12 months?
27. Did you attend school in the past 12 months?

28. If you did not attend school or work in the past 12 months, how many days in the past 12 months did your breathing problems interfere with your ability to do your regular activities?

Asthma Screening Questionnaire (ASQ)
1. Do you cough more than the average person?
2. Do you have a cough that comes mainly from your chest and not from your throat?
3. Do you have worsening of the following symptoms when you lie down to sleep?
4. Do you have worsening of the following symptoms after exercise or physical activity?
5. Do you have worsening of the following symptoms after laughing or crying?
6. Do you have worsening of the following symptoms after talking on the phone?

St. George's Respiratory Questionnaire (SGRQ)
1. Please checkmark one box to show how you describe your present health.
2. Over the past 3 months, I have cough
3. Over the past 3 months, I have brought up phlegm (sputum)
4. Over the past 3 months, I have had shortness of breath
5. Over the past 3 months, I have had attacks of wheezing
6. During the past 3 months, how many severe or very unpleasant attacks of chest problems have you had?
7. How long did the worst attack of chest problem last?
8. Over the past 3 months, in an average week, how many good days (with little chest problem) have you had?
9. If you have a wheeze, is it worse in the morning?
10. How would you describe your chest condition?
11. If you have ever had paid employment, please checkmark one of these.
12. Questions about what activities usually make you feel breathless these days:
    a. Sitting or lying still
    b. Getting washed or dressed
    c. Walking around at home
    d. Walking outside on the level
    e. Climbing up a flight of stairs
    f. Climbing hills
    g. Playing sports or games
13. Some more questions about your cough and breathlessness these days:
    a. My cough hurts
    b. My cough makes me tired
    c. I am breathless when I talk
    d. I am breathless when I bend over
    e. My cough or breathing disturbs my sleep
    f. I get exhausted easily
14. Questions about other effects that your chest problem may have on you these days:
    a. My cough or breathing is embarrassing in public
    b. My chest problem is a nuisance to my family, friends or neighbours
    c. I get afraid or panic when I cannot get my breath

d. I feel that I am not in control of my chest problem
    e. I do not expect my chest to get any better
    f. I have become frail or an invalid because of my chest
    g. Exercise is not safe for me
    h. Everything seems too much of an effort
15. Questions about your medication:
    a. My medication does not help me very much
    b. I get embarrassed using my medication in public
    c. I have unpleasant side effects from my medication
    d. My medication interferes with my life a lot
16. These are questions about how your activities might be affected by your breathing:
    a. I take a long time to get washed or dressed
    b. I cannot take a bath or shower, or I take a long time
    c. I walk slower than other people, or I stop for rests
    d. Jobs such as housework take a long time, or I have to stop for rests
    e. If I climb up one flight or stairs, I have to go slow or stop
    f. If I hurry or walk fast, I have to stop or slow down
    g. My breathing makes it difficult to do things such as climbing up hills, carrying things upstairs, light gardening such as weeding, dancing, bowling or golfing
    h. My breathing makes it difficult to do things such as carrying heavy loads, digging the garden or shovelling snow, jogging or walking at 5 kilometers per hour, playing tennis or swimming
    i. My breathing makes it difficult to things such as very heavy manual work, running, cycling, swimming fast or playing competitive sports
17. We would like to know how your chest problem usually affects your daily life:
    a. I cannot play sports or games
    b. I cannot go out for entertainment or recreation
    c. I cannot go out of the house to do the groceries
    d. I cannot do housework
    e. I cannot move far from my bed or chair
18. Please write in any other important activities that your chest problem may stop you doing.
19. Would you checkmark the box (one only) which you think best describes how your chest problem affects you?

Short Form-36 Quality of Life Questionnaire (SF-36 QoL)
1. In general, would you say your health is?
2. Compared to one year ago, how would you rate your health in general now?
3. Does your health now limit you in these activities? If so, how much?
    a. Vigorous activities, such as running, lifting heavy objects, participating in strenuous sports
    b. Moderate activities, such as moving a table, pushing a vacuum cleaner, bowling or playing golf
    c. Lifting or carrying groceries
    d. Climbing several flights of stairs

e. Climbing one flight of stairs
  f. Bending, kneeling, or stooping
  g. Walking more than a kilometer
  h. Walking several hundred meters
  i. Walking one hundred meters
  j. Bathing or dressing yourself
4. During the past 4 weeks, how much of the time have you had any of the following problems with your work or other regular activities as a result of your physical health?
  a. Cut down on the amount of time you spent on work or other activities?
  b. Accomplished less than you would like
  c. Were limited in the kind of work or other activities
  d. Had difficulty performing the work or other activities (for example, it took extra effort)
5. During the past 4 weeks, how much of the time have you had any of the following problems with your work or other regular activities as a result of any emotional problems, such as feeling depressed or anxious?
  a. Cut down on the amount of time you spent on work or other activities
  b. Accomplished less than you would like?
  c. Did work or other activities less carefully than usual
6. During the past 4 weeks, to what extent has your physical health or emotional problems interfered with your normal social activities with family, friends, neighbours, or groups?
7. How much bodily pain have you had during the past 4 weeks?
8. During the past 4 weeks, how much did pain interfere with your normal work (including both work outside the home and housework)?
9. These questions are about how you feel and how things have been with you during the past 4 weeks. For each question, please give the one answer that comes closest to the way you have been feeling. How much of the time during the past 4 weeks…?
  a. Did you feel full of life?
  b. Have you been very nervous?
  c. Have you felt so down in the dumps that nothing could cheer you up?
  d. Have you felt calm and peaceful?
  e. Did you have a lot of energy?
  f. Have you felt so downhearted and depressed?
  g. Have you been happy?
  h. Did you feel tired?
10. During the past 4 weeks, how much of the time has your physical health or emotional problems interfered with your social activities (like visiting with friends, relative, etc.)?
11. How TRUE or FALSE is each of the following statements for you?
  a. I seem to get sick a little easier than other people
  b. I am as healthy as anybody I know
  c. I expect my health to get worse
  d. My health is excellent

Work Productivity and Activity Impairment Questionnaire: General Health (WPAIGH)
  1. Are you currently employed (working for pay)?

2. During the past 7 days, how many hours did you miss from work because of your breathing problems?
3. During the past 7 days, how many hours did you miss from work because of any other reason, such as vacation, holidays, time off to participate in this study?
4. During the past 7 days, how many hours did you actually work?
5. During the past 7 days, how much did your breathing problems affect your productivity while you were working?
6. During the past 7 days, how much did your breathing affect your ability to do your regular daily activities, other than your job at work?
7. Do you currently attend classes in an academic setting?
8. During the past 7 days, how many hours did you miss from class or school because of your breathing problems?
9. During the past 7 days, how many hours did you miss from class or school because of any other reason, such as vacation, holidays, time off to participate in this study?
10. During the past 7 days, how many hours did you actually attend class or school?
11. During the past 7 days, how much did your breathing problems affect your productivity while in school or attending classes?
12. During the past 7 days, how much did your breathing problems affect your ability to do your regular daily activities, other than attending classes?

COPD Assessment Test (CAT)

On a scale of 0 to 5:
1. I never cough to I cough all the time
2. I have no phlegm (mucus) in my chest at all to My chest is completely full of phlegm
3. My chest does not feel tight at all to My chest feels very tight
4. When I walk up a hill or one flight of stairs, I am not breathless to When I walk up a hill or one flight of stairs, I am very breathless
5. I am not limited doing any activities at home to I am very limited doing activities at home
6. I am confident leaving my home despite my lung condition to I am not at all confident leaving my home because of my lung condition
7. I sleep soundly to I don't sleep soundly because of my lung condition
8. I have lots of energy to I have no energy at all

The following questionnaire was not used as a source of questions for the case-finding questionnaire because it was not completed by many UCAP subjects under the study protocol.

COPD Diagnostic Questionnaire (COPD-DQ)

1. Age in years
2. Are you now, or have you ever smoked?
3. Body mass index
4. Does the weather affect your cough?
5. Do you ever cough up phlegm from your chest when you do not have a cold?
6. Do you usually cough up phlegm first thing in the morning?
7. How frequently do you wheeze?
8. Do you have or have you had any allergies?

Appendix B – Data Collection Form

This refers to the UCAP data collection form for test-retest reliability and feedback from participants and expert reviewers.

UCAP- Undiagnosed COPD and Asthma Population Study

UCAP Questionnaire

Participant Number: ☐☐☐ — ☐☐☐

Date of Administration for Week 1: ______ / ______ / ______

1. How old are you? ☐☐

2. Are you currently smoking cigarettes or have you smoked cigarettes in the past?

☐ Yes   ☐ No

If 'yes', calculate pack years:

Average number of packs of cigarettes per day: ☐.☐☐ (20 cigarettes =1.0 pack)

Number of years spent smoking: ☐☐ (years)

Total Pack Years: ☐☐☐.☐☐ (*# packs/day x # years smoked*)

3. Are you regularly exposed to cigarette smoke (either from yourself, or from people around you) on a <u>daily</u> basis?

☐ Yes   ☐ No

4. Have you ever worked for <u>3 months or more</u> with paint, chemicals, or fumes?

☐ Yes   ☐ No

If 'yes', how many months worked? ☐☐☐☐

5. Have you ever worked for <u>3 months or more</u> with sandblasting?

☐ Yes   ☐ No

If 'yes' , how many months worked? ☐☐☐☐

UCAP Questionnaire

6. Are you currently taking the medication Salbutamol (Ventolin) for your breathing?

☐ Yes   ☐ No

7. If you have a wheeze, is it worse in the morning?

☐ Yes   ☐ No   ☐ Not applicable

8. During the past 3 months, how many severe or very unpleasant attacks of chest problems (attacks of shortness of breath or wheezing) have you had?
{Interviewer to read the responses}

☐ More than 3 attacks   ☐ 3 attacks   ☐ 2 attacks   ☐ 1 attack   ☐ No attacks

Please rate your <u>cough</u> on a scale of 0 to 5 with 0 meaning *I never cough* to 5 meaning

I cough all the time: ☐

9. Please rate your <u>sleep</u> on a scale of 0 to 5 with 0 meaning *I sleep soundly* to 5

meaning *I do not sleep soundly because of my lung condition*:   ☐

10. Please rate your <u>chest tightness</u> on a scale of 0 to 5 with 0 meaning *no chest*

tightness at all to 5 *meaning my chest feels very tight*:   ☐

11. Does your health <u>now</u> limit you in vigorous activities, such as running, lifting heavy objects, or participating in strenuous sports? *{Interviewer to read the responses}*

☐Yes, limited a lot   ☐Yes, limited a little   ☐No, not limited at all

12. How much of the time during the past 4 weeks, did you feel tired? *{Interviewer to read the responses}*

☐All of the time   ☐Most of the time   ☐Some of the time

☐A little of the time   ☐None of the time

UCAP Questionnaire

13. During the past 4 weeks, how much of the time have you had to cut down on the amount of time you spent on work or other regular activities as a result of any emotional problems, such as feeling depressed or anxious?
{Interviewer to read the responses}

☐ All of the time   ☐ Most of the time   ☐ Some of the time

☐ A little of the time   ☐ None of the time

Thank you for your time.
I will call you back in one week

UCAP Questionnaire

Participant Number: ☐☐☐ — ☐☐☐

Date of Administration for Week 2: _______ / _______ / _______

1. How old are you? ☐☐

2. Are you currently smoking cigarettes or have you smoked cigarettes in the past?

☐ Yes   ☐ No

If '**yes**', calculate pack years:

Average number of packs of cigarettes per day: ☐.☐☐ (20 cigarettes =1.0 pack)

Number of years spent smoking: ☐☐ (years)

Total Pack Years: ☐☐☐.☐☐ *(# packs/day x # years smoked)*

3. Are you regularly exposed to cigarette smoke (either from yourself, or from people around you) on a <u>daily</u> basis?

☐ Yes   ☐ No

4. Have you ever worked for <u>3 months or more</u> with paint, chemicals, or fumes?

☐ Yes   ☐ No

If 'yes', how many months worked? ☐☐☐☐

5. Have you ever worked for <u>3 months or more</u> with sandblasting?

☐ Yes   ☐ No

If 'yes', how many months worked? ☐☐☐☐

6. Are you currently taking the medication Salbutamol (Ventolin) for your breathing?

☐ Yes   ☐ No

7. If you have a wheeze, is it worse in the morning?

☐ Yes   ☐ No   ☐ Not applicable

8. During the past 3 months, how many severe or very unpleasant attacks of chest problems (attacks of shortness of breath or wheezing) have you had?
{Interviewer to read the responses}

☐ More than 3 attacks   ☐ 3 attacks   ☐ 2 attacks   ☐ 1 attack   ☐ No attacks

Please rate your <u>cough</u> on a scale of 0 to 5 with 0 meaning *I never cough* to 5 meaning *I cough all the time*: ☐

9. Please rate your <u>sleep</u> on a scale of 0 to 5 with 0 meaning *I sleep soundly* to 5 meaning *I do not sleep soundly because of my lung condition*: ☐

10. Please rate your <u>chest tightness</u> on a scale of 0 to 5 with 0 meaning *no chest tightness at all* to 5 *meaning my chest feels very tight*: ☐

11. Does your health <u>now</u> limit you in vigorous activities, such as running, lifting heavy objects, or participating in strenuous sports? *{Interviewer to read the responses}*

☐Yes, limited a lot   ☐Yes, limited a little   ☐No, not limited at all

12. How much of the time during the past 4 weeks, did you feel tired? *{Interviewer to read the responses}*

☐All of the time   ☐Most of the time   ☐Some of the time

☐A little of the time   ☐None of the time

UCAP Questionnaire

13. During the past 4 weeks, how much of the time have you had to cut down on the amount of time you spent on work or other regular activities as a result of any emotional problems, such as feeling depressed or anxious?
{Interviewer to read the responses}

☐ All of the time   ☐ Most of the time   ☐ Some of the time

☐ A little of the time   ☐ None of the time

> **Thank you for answering the UCAP Questionnaire.**
> **I will now ask you for your feedback on the questionnaire.**

1. Was the wording of the questions clear, easy to understand, and interpret?
   - ☐ Yes
   - ☐ No
   - ☐ *If no, please elaborate (i.e. what specific question and wording?):*

   ____
   ____

2. Does the list of responses for each question feel adequate?
   - ☐ Yes
   - ☐ No
   - ☐ *If no, please elaborate (i.e. what specific question and inadequacy?):*

   ____
   ____

3. How was the overall flow and structure of the questions?
   - a. Satisfactory
   - b. Not satisfactory
   - c. *If not satisfactory, please elaborate:*

   ____
   ____

4. Was the time to complete the questions reasonable?
   - a. Yes
   - b. No

5. Do you have any other comments or suggestions (*i.e.* format, wording):

   ____
   ____

Study Coordinator Section:

As the interviewer, please provide your feedback on the following questions:

1. Was the interview script clear and adequate for the interview?
   - ☐ Yes
   - ☐ No

2. Did you need to explain any questions or elaborate unduly on response options?
   - ☐ Yes If yes, which questions:_______________________________
   - ☐ No

3. Please estimate the time required to complete the questionnaire. _____ (minutes)

4. Do you have any other comments or suggestions (*i.e.* format, wording):
   ____
   ____

Appendix C – Ethics Form

 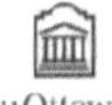 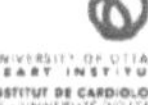

Date: 8 October 2020

To: Dr. Shawn Aaron, Ottawa Hospital Research Institute

Participating Centres:

Contact Full Name	Contact Centre
Dr. Samir Gupta	St. Michael's Hospital
Dr Chris Licskai	London Health Sciences Centre
Dr Andrew McIvor	St. Joseph's Healthcare Hamilton
Dr. Masoud Mahdavian	Royal Victoria Regional Health Centre
Dr Shawn Aaron	The Ottawa Hospital - General Campus
Dr Diane Lougheed	Kingston Health Sciences Centre (KGH Site)

CTO Project ID: 1357

Study Title: A RANDOMIZED, CONTROLLED, CLINICAL TRIAL TO ADDRESS THE BURDEN OF UNDIAGNOSED AIRFLOW OBSTRUCTION IN CANADIAN ADULTS
SHORT TITLE: UNDIAGNOSED COPD AND ASTHMA POPULATION STUDY (UCAP)

Study Sponsor: Ottawa Hospital Research Institute

Application Type: Provincial Amendment Form

Amendment Reference/ID: Protocol Amendment 4.0

Review Type: Delegated

Date Approval Issued: 08/Oct/2020

Study Approval Expiry Date: 24/Jan/2021

____

Dear Provincial Applicant,

The OHSN-REB (General Campus Panel) has reviewed the amendment to the study and granted approval as of the date noted above. This approval applies to all participating centres (listed above) that have received ethics approval to conduct the study.

Provincial documents approved:

Document Name	Document Date	Document Version
Screening Telephone Worksheet Case Finding Study	18/Sep/2020	
Protocol Version 4	28/Sep/2020	
English Oral Consent Update Information with Questionnaire	06/Oct/2020	

REB members involved in the research project do not participate in the review, discussion or decision.

OHSN-REB (General Campus Panel) operates in compliance with, and is constituted in accordance with, the requirements of the Tri-Council Policy Statement: Ethical Conduct for Research Involving Humans (TCPS 2); the International Conference on Harmonisation Good Clinical Practice Consolidated Guideline (ICH GCP); Part C, Division 5 of the Food and Drug Regulations; Part 4 of the Natural Health Products Regulations; Part 3 of the Medical Devices Regulations and the provisions of the Ontario Personal Health Information Protection Act (PHIPA 2004) and its applicable regulations. OHSN-REB (General Campus Panel) is qualified through the CTO REB Qualification Program and is registered with the U.S. Department of Health and Human Services (DHHS) Office for Human Research Protection (OHRP).

Please do not hesitate to contact us if you have any questions.

Sincerely,

87

Appendix D – List of Predictors and Associated Level of Significance

The following appendix outlines the results of the univariate statistical association to the multinomial outcome. These were conducted as a preliminary investigation to determine their potential for inclusion in the pool of candidate predictors. Complementary considerations for inclusion and exclusion were clinical relevance and usefulness, and similarities to other questions. Tables C1-C6 shows the question with the corresponding p-value, inclusion or exclusion verdict, and the missing count.

Table D1. List of Predictors and Associated Level of Significance for Asthma Screening Questionnaire (ASQ)

ASQ	p-value	Included/Excluded	Missing (n)
Do you cough more than the average person?	0.629	Excluded	9
Do you have a cough that comes mainly from your chest and not from your throat?	**0.068***	Excluded	13
Do you have worsening of the following symptoms when you lie down to sleep?			
• Cough	**0.227***	Included	25
• Chest tightness	**0.002***	Included	32
• Wheeze	**0.040***	Included	25
• Short of breath	**0.050***	Excluded; collinearity	26
Do you have worsening of the following symptoms after exercise or physical activity?			
• Cough	0.461	Excluded	25
• Chest tightness	**0.066***	Included	26
• Wheeze	**0.144***	Included	25
• Short of breath	**0.003***	Included	16
Do you have worsening of the following symptoms after laughing or crying?			
• Cough	**0.002***	Included	27
• Chest tightness	**0.152***	Included	38
• Wheeze	**0.186***	Included	35
• Short of breath	0.911	Excluded	33
Do you have worsening of the following symptoms after talking on the phone?			
• Cough	**0.237***	Excluded	37

	0.343	Excluded	41
• Chest tightness	0.261	Excluded	40
• Wheeze	0.770	Excluded	34
• Short of breath			

Level of significance: *p-value <0.25

Table D2. List of Predictors and Associated Level of Significance for Personal Information Sheet

Personal Information Sheet	p-value	Included/Excluded	Missing (n)
Age, years	**0.000***	Included	0
Sex	**0.000***	Included	0
Race	**0.026***	Excluded	1
Education	**0.050***	Excluded	0
Income	**0.022***	Excluded	0
Have you ever worked for 3 months or more at any of the following occupations: hard-rock mining, coal mining, sandblasting, working with asbestos, chemical or plastics manufacturing, flour, feed or grain milling, cotton or jute processing, foundry or steel milling, welding, firefighting, farming, forestry, saw-milling, work with paint, chemicals, or fumes	**0.000***	Included: Sandblasting and Paint, chemicals, fumes; potential risk factor for adult asthma[162,163]	0
Are you regularly exposed to any of the following daily? • Smoking (primary or second-hand) • Pets (dogs, cats, or fur animals)	**0.000*** 0.913	Included[22, 28] Excluded	40 39
Are you currently smoking cigarettes?	**0.000***	Included	0
Have you every smoked pot/marijuana?	**0.231***	Included; potential risk factor[173]	4
Have you ever tried an electronic cigarette, also known as an e-cigarette?	0.310	Excluded	89
The last time you used an e-cigarette, did it contain nicotine?	**0.047***	Excluded; high number of missing	1,345
Do you have a family doctor?	0.797	Excluded	45

Question	p-value	Decision	Missing
Can you see your family doctor within a week of requesting an appointment?	0.840	Excluded	45
What is the distance in kms from your home to your family doctor?	0.745	Excluded	45
Did any doctor give you an alternative diagnosis for your respiratory symptoms?	N/A	Excluded	1,302
Did any doctor refer you to a specialist for your respiratory symptoms?	0.441	Excluded	0
Did you ever have any of the following procedures for your respiratory symptoms?	0.366	Excluded	0
In the past 12 months, did you visit your general practitioner or a nurse practitioner or another physician at a walk-in clinic for any breathing problems?	0.409	Excluded	9
In the past 12 months, did you visit an emergency practitioner or a nurse practitioner or another physician at a walk-in clinic for any breathing problem?	0.385	Excluded	13
In the past 12 months, did you visit an emergency department for any breathing problems?	N/A	Excluded	13
In the past 12 months, were you hospitalized for any breathing problems or respiratory illness?	**0.050***	Included	18
Are you currently taking any medications for your breathing? Ventolin	**0.005***	Included	0
Did you work in the past 12 months?	**0.002***	Excluded; no clinical relevance	13
Did you attend school in the past 12 months?	0.298	Excluded	22
If you did not attend school or work in the past 12 months, how many days in the past 12 months did your breathing problems interfere with your ability to do your regular activities?	0.258	Excluded	13

Level of significance: *p-value <0.25

Table D3. List of Predictors and Associated Level of Significance for COPD Assessment Test (CAT)

CAT	p-value	Included/Excluded	Missing (n)
I never cough to I cough all the time	0.318	Relevant predictor for OLD – Included	5
I have no phlegm (mucus) in my chest at all to My chest is completely full of phlegm	**0.047***	Included	5
My chest does not feel tight at all to My chest feels very tight	**0.091***	Included	5
When I walk up a hill or one flight of stairs I am not breathless to When I walk up a hill or one flight of stairs I am very breathless	**0.127***	Excluded; collinearity	7
I am not limited doing any activities at home to I am very limited doing activities at home	**0.106***	Excluded; collinearity	8
I am confident leaving my home despite my lung condition to I am not at all confident leaving my home because of my lung condition	**0.185***	Included	8
I sleep soundly to I don't sleep soundly because of my lung condition	**0.136***	Included	7
I have lots of energy to I have no energy at all	0.760	Excluded	5

Level of significance: *p-value <0.25

Table D4. List of Predictors and Associated Level of Significance for St. George's Respiratory Questionnaire (SGRQ)

SGRQ	p-value	Included/Excluded	Missing (n)
Over the past 3 months, I have coughed	0.683	Excluded	2
Over the past 3 months, I have brought up phlegm (sputum)	**0.198***	Excluded; collinearity	5
Over the past 3 months, I have had shortness of breath	**0.047***	Included	6
Over the past 3 months, I have had attacks of wheezing	**0.000***	Excluded; collinearity	10

During the past 3 months, how many severe or very unpleasant attacks of chest problems have you had?	**0.014***	Included	3
How long did the worst attack of chest problem last?	0.375	Excluded	1
Over the past 3 months, in an average week, how many good days (with little chest problem) have you had?	**0.242***	Excluded; similarity to question 5	13
If you have a wheeze, is it worse in the morning?	**0.000***	Included	32
How would you describe your chest condition?	0.812	Excluded	2
Questions about what activities usually make you feel breathless these days:			
• Sitting or lying still	**0.005***	Included	33
• Getting washed or dressed	0.255	Excluded	26
• Walking around at home	0.625	Excluded	26
• Walking outside on the level	**0.174***	Excluded; collinearity	29
• Climbing up a flight of stairs	**0.042***	Excluded; collinearity	12
• Climbing hills	**0.030***	Excluded; collinearity	11
• Playing sports or games	0.453	Excluded	45
Some more questions about your cough and breathlessness these days:			
• My cough hurts	**0.013***	Included	21
• My cough makes me tired	**0.048***	Excluded; collinearity	20
• I am breathless when I talk	0.405	Excluded	23
• I am breathless when I bend over	0.342	Excluded	28
• My cough or breathing disturbs my sleep	**0.072***	Excluded; collinearity	19
• I get exhausted easily	0.626	Excluded	23
Questions about other effects that your chest problem may have on you these days:			
• My cough or breathing is embarrassing in public	0.471	Excluded	10
• My chest problem is a nuisance to my family, friends or neighbours	0.610	Excluded	13
• I get afraid or panic when I cannot get my breath	**0.147***	Excluded	14
• I feel that I am not in control of my chest problem	**0.079***	Included	17

• I do not expect my chest to get any better	**0.025***	Excluded; collinearity	20
• I have become frail or an invalid because of my chest	0.488	Excluded	15
• Exercise is not safe for me	0.245	Excluded	19
• Everything seems too much of an effort	0.352	Excluded	19
Questions about your medication:			
• My medication does not help me very much	N/A	Excluded	1,180
• I get embarrassed using my medication in public	N/A	Excluded	1,184
• I have unpleasant side effects from my medication	N/A	Excluded	1,184
• My medication interferes with my life a lot	N/A	Excluded	1,186
These are questions about how your activities might be affected by your breathing:			
• I take a long time to get washed or dressed	0.622	Excluded	8
• I cannot take a bath or shower, or I take a long time	**0.022***	Excluded	11
• I walk slower than other people, or I stop for rests	0.402	Excluded	10
• Jobs such as housework take a long time, or I have to stop for rests	0.355	Excluded	7
• If I climb up one flight or stairs, I have to go slow or stop	**0.062***	Included	8
• If I hurry or walk fast, I have to stop or slow down	**0.076***	Included	13
• My breathing makes it difficult to do things such as climbing up hills, carrying things upstairs, light gardening such as weeding, dancing, bowling or golfing	**0.001***	Excluded; collinearity	7
• My breathing makes it difficult to do things such as carrying heavy loads, digging the garden or shoveling snow, jogging or walking at 5 kilometers per	**0.004***	Excluded; collinearity	13

	0.016*	Excluded; collinearity	13
hour, playing tennis or swimming			
• My breathing makes it difficult to things such as very heavy manual work, running, cycling, swimming fast or playing competitive sports	0.016*	Excluded; collinearity	13
We would like to know how your chest problem usually affects your daily life:			
• I cannot play sports or games	0.263	Excluded	12
• I cannot go out for entertainment or recreation	0.916	Excluded	12
• I cannot go out of the house to do the groceries	0.931	Excluded	9
• I cannot do housework	0.907	Excluded	9
• I cannot move far from my bed or chair	0.310	Excluded	13
Please write in any other important activities that your chest problem may stop you doing.	N/A	Excluded; written responses and high missing count	1,084
Would you checkmark the box (one only) which you think best describes how your chest problem affects you?	N/A	Excluded	11

Level of significance: *p-value <0.25

Table D5. List of Predictors and Associated Level of Significance for Short Form-36 Quality of Life Questionnaire (SF-36 QoL)

SF-36 QoL	p-value	Included/Excluded	Missing (n)
In general, would you say your health is?	N/A	Excluded	4
Compared to one year ago, how would you rate your health in general now?	N/A	Excluded	5
Does your health now limit you in these activities? If so, how much?			
• Vigorous activities, such as running, lifting heavy objects, participating in strenuous sports	0.000*	Included	10
• Moderate activities, such as moving a table, pushing a	0.002*	Included	11

vacuum cleaner, bowling or playing golf			
• Lifting or carrying groceries	0.264	Excluded	11
• Climbing several flights of stairs	**0.012***	Excluded; collinearity	10
• Climbing one flight of stairs	**0.028***	Excluded; collinearity	9
• Bending, kneeling, or stooping	0.528	Excluded	8
• Walking more than a kilometer	**0.072***	Included	12
• Walking several hundred meters	**0.207***	Excluded; collinearity	10
• Walking one hundred meters	**0.066***	Excluded; collinearity	11
• Bathing or dressing yourself	0.847	Excluded	9
During the past 4 weeks, how much of the time have you had any of the following problems with your work or other regular activities as a result of your physical health?			
• Cut down on the amount of time you spent on work or other activities?	0.906	Excluded	11
• Accomplished less than you would like	0.964	Excluded	7
• Were limited in the kind of work or other activities	**0.123***	Excluded; shares similarity to physical activity questions	6
• Had difficulty performing the work or other activities (for example, it took extra effort)	0.922	Excluded	6
During the past 4 weeks, how much of the time have you had any of the following problems with your work or other regular activities as a result of any emotional problems, such as feeling depressed or anxious?			
• Cut down on the amount of time you spent on work or other activities	**0.227***	Included[160,161,161,161,161]	5
• Accomplished less than you would like?	0.380	Excluded	5
• Did work or other activities less carefully than usual	0.694	Excluded	5
During the past 4 weeks, to what extent has your physical health or emotional problems interfered with your normal social activities with family, friends, neighbours, or groups?	0.313	Excluded	7

	p-value	Included/Excluded	Missing (n)
How much bodily pain have you had during the past 4 weeks?	0.392	Excluded - based on clinical judgement	8
During the past 4 weeks, how much did pain interfere with your normal work (including both work outside the home and housework)?	**0.068***	Excluded – based on clinical judgement	9
How much of the time during the past 4 weeks…?	0.692		10
• Did you feel full of life?		Excluded	
• Have you been very nervous?	0.585	Excluded	8
• Have you felt so down in the dumps that nothing could cheer you up?	0.433	Excluded	8
• Have you felt calm and peaceful?	0.488	Excluded	8
• Did you have a lot of energy?	0.712	Excluded	6
• Have you felt so downhearted and depressed?	0.353	Excluded	8
• Have you been happy?	**0.249***	Included; relevant	8
• Did you feel worn out?	**0.153***	Included	6
• Did you feel tired?	**0.052***	Included	8
During the past 4 weeks, how much of the time has your physical health or emotional problems interfered with social activities?	0.729	Excluded	13
How TRUE or FALSE is each of the following statements for you?			
• I seem to get sick a little easier than other people	**0.149***	Excluded; no clinical relevance	9
• I am as healthy as anybody I know		Excluded	8
• I expect my health to get worse	0.855	Excluded	8
• My health is excellent	0.630	0.630	7

Level of significance: *p-value <0.25

Table D6. List of Predictors and Associated Level of Significance for Work Productivity and Activity Impairment Questionnaire (WPAIGH)

Work Productivity and Activity Impairment Questionnaire: General Health	p-value	Included/Excluded	Missing (n)
Are you currently employed (working for pay)?	**0.003***	Excluded; no clinical relevance	7

During the past 7 days, how many hours did you miss from work because of your breathing problems?	**0.038***	Included	13
During the past 7 days, how many hours did you miss from work because of any other reason, such as vacation, holidays, time off to participate in this study?	0.4163	Excluded	15
During the past 7 days, how many hours did you actually work?	**0.008***	Excluded; no clinical relevance	13
During the past 7 days, how much did your breathing problems affect your productivity while you were working?	**0.011***	Included	12
During the past 7 days, how much did your breathing affect your ability to do your regular daily activities, other than your job at work?	**0.156***	Excluded; similar to previous activity limitation questions	10
Do you currently attend classes in an academic setting?	0.656	Excluded	10
During the past 7 days, how many hours did you miss from class or school because of your breathing problems?	0.959	Excluded	10
During the past 7 days, how many hours did you miss from class or school because of any other reason, such as vacation, holidays, time off to participate in this study?	0.960	Excluded	10
During the past 7 days, how many hours did you actually attend class or school?	**0.246***	Excluded; no clinical relevance	10
During the past 7 days, how much did your breathing problems affect your productivity while in school or attending classes?	0.903	Excluded	10
During the past 7 days, how much did your breathing problems affect your ability to do your regular daily activities, other than attending classes?	0.904	Excluded	10

Level of significance: *p-value <0.25